Praise for *The Tapping Solution f*

"I've spent years teaching people around the world about
the power of choice, and the power of action. If you're in chronic pain,
I suggest you choose this book, and follow the program inside. Nick's results with
helping people relieve chronic pain speak for themselves. It's that simple."

— **Tony Robbins**, author of #1 *New York Times* bestseller *MONEY Master the Game*

"Chronic pain has reached epidemic proportions in the United States—
often leading to lifelong addiction to pain medication. But there's another way
to deal with it. Safely, naturally, and effectively. And that is the good news offered
in Nick Ortner's latest book, *The Tapping Solution for Pain Relief*. It's a winner."

— **Christiane Northrup, M.D.**, author of *Women's Bodies, Women's Wisdom*

"Put away your skepticism; this really works. I have worked with
Nick and had great results with tapping in my own life."

— **Dr. Wayne W. Dyer**, author of *Wishes Fulfilled*

"I believe Nick Ortner's teachings are easy to use and practical
but work like magic. He certainly has taught me to magically release
or dissolve problems of all sorts through the process of tapping."

— **Louise Hay**, author of *You Can Heal Your Life*

"If you're living with chronic pain and all the stress and exhaustion it brings, turn to Nick
Ortner. There's no better person to guide you towards relief. I've personally experienced the
profound benefits of tapping and I know this simple tool can help you, too. Try this method today. You have nothing to lose! A life filled with health and possibilities awaits you."

— **Kris Carr**, *New York Times* best-selling author of *Crazy Sexy Kitchen*

"If you struggle with chronic pain, and sometimes feel desperate for relief, you've probably
encountered plenty of 'solutions' that simply don't work. But, in *The Tapping Solution for
Pain Relief*, Nick Ortner provides an accessible framework for understanding the connection
between body, emotions, and stress that can create pain. I've found his practical, easy-to-
follow techniques to be an important breakthrough in the field of mind-body medicine."

— **Ruth Buczynski, Ph.D.**, licensed psychologist,
president of The National Institute for the Clinical Application of Behavioral Medicine

"A spectacular resource for immediately reversing pain symptoms. *So* important in an environment where our emergency rooms and medical clinics are overcrowded. Finally, a book that empowers patients to heal! When patients get a hold of this, it will change our entire medical system."

— **Kim D'Eramo, D.O.**, board-certified emergency physician

"Pain is nature's most vivid way of telling you what not to do. Chronic pain, however, no longer serves that useful function, yet 1.5 billion people worldwide suffer with it. They also spend billions and billions of dollars every year on medications that are either futile or that dull not only the pain but also their ability to think and function at their peak. This book presents something new, natural, and effective for those 1.5 billion souls. Many will find it a godsend."

— **David Feinstein, Ph.D.**, co-author of *The Promise of Energy Psychology*

"If you or a loved one is in pain, you need this book. In clear yet medically accurate language, Nick Ortner explains the many puzzles of pain—it's not always linked to a diagnosis and often resists conventional solutions. Using vivid and compelling case histories of pain sufferers, as well as the latest research, he illuminates the emotional problems and subconscious patterns that exacerbate pain. He shows how to use the novel technique of acupoint tapping to relieve both chronic and acute pain. Tapping scripts for common pain problems make the techniques even more accessible. The take-home message of this book is that you don't have to continue suffering; a quick and simple solution is as close as your fingertips."

— **Dawson Church, Ph.D.**,
best-selling author of the award-winning book *The Genie in Your Genes*

"*The Tapping Solution for Pain Relief* is full of simple, highly effective techniques for reducing and eliminating many chronic ailments. It's amazing to think that by literally 'tapping' into the power of the mind you can completely rid your body of physical pain. The research is clear and compelling and Nick Ortner does an excellent job of teaching us how to unlock this hidden healing potential. This book is a must read for anyone who wants to heal their body, safely, naturally, and permanently. I can't recommend it highly enough"

— **Jon Gabriel**, international best-selling author
and creator of *The Gabriel Method* and *Visualization for Weight Loss*

"Pain is the most common symptom telling us that there is a problem, which may be physical, mental, chemical, and/or emotional. In this brilliant book, Nick takes on all the causes and offers you one of the easiest and most effective tools for living a pain-free life!"

— **C. Norman Shealy, M.D., Ph.D.**,
CEO, National Institute of Holistic Medicine and author of *Living Bliss*

"If you're struggling with chronic pain, this book is a powerful first step in a successful journey toward a pain-free life. Nick has helped thousands of people get the pain relief they¹ve been searching for, and you can be next."

— **Jack Canfield**

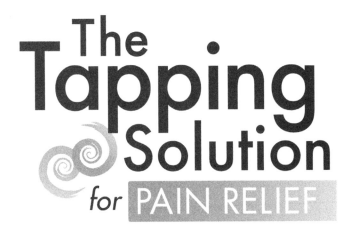

The Tapping Solution
for PAIN RELIEF

ALSO BY NICK ORTNER

The Tapping Solution: A Revolutionary System for Stress-Free Living

The above title is available at your local bookstore or may be ordered by visiting:

Hay House USA: www.hayhouse.com®
Hay House Australia: www.hayhouse.com.au
Hay House UK: www.hayhouse.co.uk
Hay House India: www.hayhouse.co.in

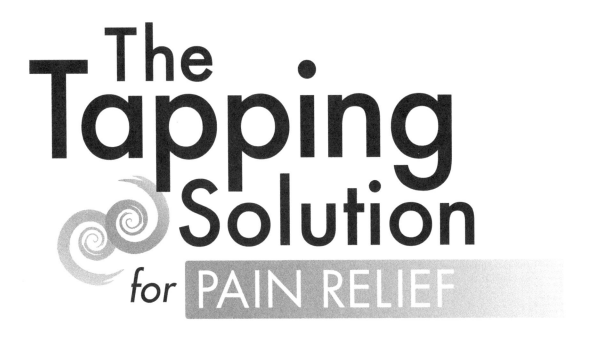

The Tapping Solution
for PAIN RELIEF

A STEP-BY-STEP GUIDE TO REDUCING AND ELIMINATING CHRONIC PAIN

NICK ORTNER

HAY HOUSE, INC.
Carlsbad, California • New York City
London • Sydney • New Delhi

Published in the United States by: Hay House, Inc.: www.hayhouse.com® • **Published in Australia by:** Hay House Australia Pty. Ltd.: www.hayhouse.com.au • **Published in the United Kingdom by:** Hay House UK, Ltd.: www.hayhouse.co.uk • **Published in India by:** Hay House Publishers India: www.hayhouse.co.in

Cover design: Michelle Polizzi
Interior design: Riann Bender
X-ray images and Tapping Points Illustration: Courtesy of the author
Tapping Tree Illustration: © 2012 Rachelle Meyer - www.rachellemeyer.com

Library of Congress Cataloging-in-Publication Data for the original edition

Ortner, Nick
  The tapping solution for pain relief : a step-by-step guide to reducing and eliminating chronic pain / Nick Ortner. -- 1st edition.
      pages cm
    ISBN 978-1-4019-4524-4 (hardback)
  1. Emotional Freedom Techniques. 2. Chronic pain--Treatment. 3. Mind and body therapies. I. Title.
  RC489.E45O782 2015
  616'.0472--dc23
                    2014034165

Tradepaper ISBN: 978-1-4019-4525-1

12 11 10 9 8 7 6 5 4 3
1st edition, April 2015
2nd edition, September 2016

Printed in the United States of America

*To the reader: may this book provide you
with the pain relief you most desire and deserve.*

CONTENTS

FOREWORD

Throughout my years practicing as a board-certified urologist and pain expert, I've become known within the medical community as the guy who can treat the "impossible" chronic pain cases. One 50-year-old patient was referred to me after he spent years suffering from chronic pain that no one else could resolve. Another, just 33 years old, was in so much pain that she could barely walk. Yet another, a 41-year-old woman, had so much nerve pain that attending to her most basic needs took all of her time and energy.

Each of these people came to my office with a vague hope of getting some minor relief, and they were all amazed to walk out pain-free—or at least dramatically improved. They were downright thrilled weeks and months later when they continued to experience little to no pain.

I never could have helped these patients (and countless others like them) without tapping. I say this with absolute confidence because I've had so many opportunities to use this technique with patients on a daily basis. Over the past 15 years, I've witnessed the incredible pain-relief results that tapping can produce. And it's not just me; when comparing medical providers who use tapping to those who don't, it's as if we are playing chess while everyone else is playing checkers.

So why does tapping work so well to relieve pain? As I have come to realize, chronic, unremitting pain is often tied to unresolved emotional issues. As you'll see in this book, the current medical literature supports this. We know the physical pain is real, but the physiological mechanisms that magnify and perpetuate it are exaggerated by the presence of unresolved negative emotions, which may be the result of experiences far in your past or more recent emotional turmoil. Let me explain.

On the physiological plane, there are typically two main mechanisms involved in chronic pain. First, there is chronic tension and spasm of the muscles. As these muscles tense up, there is less blood supply and lower oxygen levels in the muscle tissue, and that causes a great deal of pain. The second physiological mechanism causing chronic pain is hypersensitivity of the nerves. When people are in a chronic fight-or-flight state, stress hormones are released, and those hormones have a huge influence in sensitizing nerves. When the nerves are sensitized, everything just hurts more. The way that we think and feel about our pain can also influence the sensitization of nerves because our general anxiety leads to the release of more stress hormones, and the cycle perpetuates.

The other thing to take into account is that we all have the innate ability to heal—even when it comes to finding relief from chronic pain. However, as Dr. Bruce Lipton's work has shown, when the body is in a stress state, the cells go into protection/survival mode. This means that the body heals more slowly when we are stressed. Only when the body comes out of that stress state do the cells return to healing and regeneration mode, which is when lasting pain relief becomes possible.

Tapping is so effective at relieving chronic pain because it helps patients release the unresolved emotions that are keeping the body in a stressed-out state. By tapping to remove the negative emotional charge from specific events and other past and current issues, the brain gets the message that it is safe to relax tense muscles and lessen nerve sensitivity. That's when the body can heal itself—of chronic pain and other symptoms as well.

While my expertise is in treating chronic pelvic pain, the basic underlying physiological mechanisms that cause pain can be applied to pain anywhere in the body.

There are untold millions of people around the world suffering from chronic pain every day and the need for help is so great that I was thrilled when Nick told me that he was writing this book. Tapping is a game changer when it comes to getting relief from chronic pain, and Nick has such a wonderful way of explaining complex topics very simply and in plain English that I'm certain many will find the help they're looking for.

This book leads you through a powerful, effective process to relieve chronic pain for good. I urge you to dive into this process, however "weird" it may seem at first, with your full commitment. It targets what is often the true source of your pain—your emotions, your stress, your traumas. Once you release those, your body's innate ability to heal itself will take over. Like thousands of others, you'll be blown away by the pain-relief results you experience.

Eric Robins, M.D.

INTRODUCTION

If you've started reading this book, it's likely because you or someone you love is experiencing physical pain and you're looking for a solution. And if you're like most people who experience chronic pain, you're probably frustrated, angry, disappointed, or even depressed.

I get it. Pain isn't fun. The physical experience of pain ranges from unpleasant to excruciating and torturous. The emotional experience that comes with it can be just as bad, especially when the physical pain is chronic.

Pain often limits us in startling ways, from what we can do to where we can go, how we interact with others, what we're able to create in the world, and how we show up on a daily basis. And as the pain wears on, it wears us down. Over time, we start to feel as if we can't bounce back. We keep searching for a solution—for lasting pain relief—but nothing makes the pain go away for good.

Here are just some of the things I hear when I work with people who have chronic pain:

> "The pain is constant; it never stops. I take Advil like it's PEZ Candy just so I can function, but it never goes away."

> "I fell about ten years ago and had a traumatic foot injury. I've had six surgeries on my foot . . . the pain is still excruciating. I've tried everything, and nothing helps. The surgeries have only made my pain worse, and I'm just so angry about it."

"I've tried to be tough, but . . . the pain in my back, it just goes up and down, and it won't stop."

If any of this sounds familiar, you're not alone. More than 100 million Americans suffer from chronic pain, and that's just a small sampling of the number of people suffering around the world. Every time I speak onstage, regardless of what continent I'm on, I ask who in the audience is experiencing chronic pain. Without fail, at least one-third of the people in the audience raise their hands. And none of these events is focused on physical pain or pain relief!

In Western culture, the normal "solutions" we've been taught to seek out are doctors, surgeries, injections, and medications. All of that has its place, but when it comes to chronic pain, what I hear repeatedly is that conventional medicine isn't getting the job done. The best we can hope for from pain pills, injections, and even surgery is a reduction in pain or some temporary numbing. Often, though, those benefits also come with unwanted side effects, which only increases the emotional pain.

It's an ongoing cycle of physical and emotional pain that so many people get stuck in.

Let me be clear that this isn't a doctor-bashing book or a book that says Western medicine is wrong. It's just the opposite. It's a book that suggests a way for Eastern and Western medicine to work together, to complement each other, and to provide the lasting pain relief and healing you deserve.

This book presents a startling alternative, an option that, at first glance, may seem silly and strange but very quickly reveals its power. Tapping, also known as Emotional Freedom Techniques, or EFT, is a tool I've spent the last ten years using, teaching, and spreading to every corner of the globe I can. It blends Eastern acupressure with Western psychology, allowing you to address deeper emotions that can contribute to pain. The relief it provides for physical pain, as well as stress and much more, is simply incredible.

I began my own tapping journey in 2004, when I got pain relief in minutes while tapping on neck pain from a "crick" in my neck that I'd woken up with that morning. I was amazed at how quickly I got results. I'd had that kind of pain before and had always had to wait it out, which meant spending a few days experiencing nonstop pain and stiffness in my neck, shoulders, and upper back. But this time, because of tapping, the pain and discomfort vanished within minutes, and I was able to go through my day comfortably pain-free. I remember thinking,

Wow, this tapping thing really works! Soon after, I began teaching tapping to friends and family, and I saw them get similar results.

Before long, I came up with what then seemed like a crazy idea—to make a documentary about tapping. It was such a powerful tool; I knew I had to share it with as many people as possible. I had zero filmmaking experience and had to max out credit cards to pay for it, but, in the end, the film I made with my sister, Jessica Ortner, and my good friend Nick Polizzi was the start of a new life for me.

Ever since making that documentary, *The Tapping Solution,* I've been help-ing people around the world get pain relief and create the lives they've always dreamed of living. It has all come from tapping, and it all began with the four-day tapping retreat we hosted and filmed back in 2007.

During that retreat, we worked with ten people, all handpicked from the hun-dreds of applications we received. One of the participants was Jodi. When we first met her at her home in Texas, she'd been living with chronic pain from fibromy-algia for 15 years. Most of her pain was in her knees, and it got so bad that she would resort to crawling around her house, unable to withstand any more agony from walking. During a typical night, her pain would wake her up repeatedly, as much as 20 times!

In the first few minutes of talking to Jodi, I learned two things about her. First, she'd lived through several traumatic experiences as a young girl, including seeing her father beat her mother. Second, even on her worst days, she was determined to stay positive and productive. In spite of the incredible pain she was living with, Jodi was a teacher, healer, mother of four, wife, and aspiring author, and she was committed to taking her life—her health as well as her writing—to the next level.

During the first day of the retreat, we explored what had been happening in her life when her knee pain began. She shared that her daughter had been diag-nosed with HIV and had also become pregnant at that time. She described that period of time as "sad," which prompted Rick Wilkes, the EFT practitioner who was working with her, to dub hers "sad knees."

After tapping through her sadness that she hadn't been able to save her daugh-ter from those experiences, Jodi was able to walk up and down stairs without ex-periencing any pain. Afraid to believe in the possibility of lasting pain relief, she at first assumed it was one of those rare times when her pain would disappear for a short while only to return with a vengeance. By the second day of the re-treat, though, for the first time in many years, she could easily do the long nature walks she'd always loved but had had to give up because of her knee pain. In fact, without even realizing it, Jodi found herself walking ahead of the entire group! It was the first time in a long time that Jodi had allowed herself to believe that she was finally, after all those years, pain-free.

Within the months that followed the retreat, she continued to tap daily, sometimes several times a day, and was regularly sleeping through the night. Each morning, she woke up refreshed and ready to start her day—and amazed by how good she felt! Because her knee pain was gone, she could easily walk up and down stairs, so her husband began building them their dream home—a *two-story* home. Jodi was also hiking regularly again and had written two books within a two-month period after years of not being able to complete a single one! Her relationships with her family had even improved.

Just as important, Jodi had made some other significant changes in her life. During the retreat, when she was tapping on her "sad knees," she'd acknowledged her habit of taking care of everyone around her but not taking time to care for herself. After the retreat, in addition to tapping daily, Jodi made a point of taking the time to slow down, listen to her body, and take better care of herself.

In 2014, nearly seven years after that retreat, I caught up with Jodi and was thrilled to hear about her new life. She still taps every day, and she continues to be pain-free. "Since the retreat, I've only lived in two-story houses," she shared, "so I'm up and down the stairs all day long." She now has a thriving business as an EFT practitioner and has also had success as a writer and speaker.

Throughout this book you'll meet more people like Jodi—Cathy, Bobbie, Nancy, Vickie, and Thomas. Like Jodi, each of them began this tapping journey feeling imprisoned by their chronic pain. After tapping through the issues beneath their pain, all of them—and many others—could finally, once again, live pain-free and begin stepping into the life they'd always dreamed of.

In addition to all of this experienced evidence, I'll also share recent scientific findings that explain the power of tapping: why the pain is happening, how the pain is affected by emotions and stress, and why tapping may be so effective at relieving the pain.

After we learn how to tap in Chapter 2, we'll begin the pain-relief journey by looking at the relationship between stress and pain in Chapter 3. Then in Chapter 4 we'll revisit what happened when the pain began.

Next we'll explore the impact of your diagnosis in Chapter 5. You can skip this chapter if you don't have a diagnosis, although I always recommend getting a diagnosis from the doctor before relying on tapping for pain relief. It's important to know what is happening in your body first and foremost, and then use tapping to get rid of the pain.

After exploring your diagnosis, we'll process and release unresolved emotions in Chapter 6.

People are often amazed by how deeply intertwined their life experiences are with their pain, which is why we'll explore one of the most significant parts of your past, your childhood, in Chapter 7. Even if you had a happy childhood, I urge you to complete this chapter. Seemingly small and insignificant experiences can get lodged in the body long after they happen, and years later they can contribute to chronic pain.

In Chapter 8, we'll explore how we, as humans, tend to resist change, even positive ones like pain relief. We'll also take a look at the deeper meaning of your pain and any messages your body may be trying to send you through this pain.

In Chapter 9, you'll begin to create a new relationship with your body, yourself, and your life. Then, as you continue moving toward a pain-free life, you'll create a new vision for your future in Chapter 10. As you'll discover, that vision will need to include, but also extend beyond, physical pain relief.

Throughout the journey, I'll guide you through tapping scripts and ask you to complete exercises to help you discover the deeper sources of your chronic pain. If you want results, it's important that you do these exercises, as well as the tapping. This process works, but only if you follow it. I've guided thousands of people through it and seen many of them dive in and get the pain relief they so desperately wanted. Do yourself the favor of making this book and this process a new priority in your life. Complete all the exercises and, above all, do the tapping every day and as often as you can.

For most of the exercises in the book, I'll ask you to record your experiences in a journal that you use exclusively for this process. This is really important; by keeping all your tapping notes and journal entries in one place, you'll get a clearer and more complete picture of the issues related to your pain. As you'll see, assembling these layers and tapping through them is critical for pain relief.

This process is different for everyone, but for most it requires a unique blend of thinking big and small at the same time. Our ultimate goal, of course, is pain relief. That's the big picture. To get there, you'll need to stay tuned in to the little shifts you experience on a moment-to-moment, day-to-day basis. By noticing those smaller changes in your pain, your emotions, your beliefs, and your body, you'll get better results. Through the tapping, you'll also experience stress relief that will make you feel better physically and emotionally.

After all these years doing this work, the pain relief people get by using this process still inspires and amazes me. It always feels like a miracle to them, and it often does to me as well! Although this process is backed by solid science, as you do the tapping, you should also let yourself believe in miracles. Get excited when your pain lessens even a little bit. Every change, whether big or small, counts. Let yourself celebrate each one.

What you'll find as you use this process is that tapping is not just a technique to relieve pain and help your body heal. It's an incredibly powerful tool that, again and again, changes people's lives. As you explore the deeper source of your pain, you'll have the opportunity to heal the pain in your body, as well as the emotional pain that has made its mark on your life. Through that, you'll see how deeply interconnected everything is and how true transformation really is possible.

Start right now by envisioning your life without this pain. Imagine waking up to a pain-free day. Picture yourself enjoying the activities you once loved to do but haven't done lately because of your pain. Find that sliver of hope that maybe there is an answer. Then turn the page and begin tapping your way toward a pain-free life. I've seen it happen firsthand for thousands of people, and far more people than that have experienced that pain relief for themselves. Now it's your turn.

CHAPTER 1

THE SCIENCE OF PAIN

It was a quiet Sunday morning, and I'd just sat down to enjoy my coffee and scan the news. I didn't expect to be blown away by the first headline I saw from *The New York Times:*

DOCTORS IDENTIFY A NEW KNEE LIGAMENT

Come again? I was reading this headline in late 2013, a time in history when we were supposed to have unlocked the secrets of the human body, and they'd just discovered a "new" ligament! This wasn't a new gene or surgical process; it wasn't a breakthrough drug or an unknown chemical in the body. It was a simple ligament! That's even more shocking when you consider that 600,000 knee-replacement surgeries are performed each year in the United States—we've certainly spent a lot of time looking at knees and ligaments. As that headline clearly demonstrates, though, we're still discovering new parts of the knee.

While the headline made me laugh, it's also a powerful reminder of how little we know about the human body, about its many components, why it does what it does, and how we can heal it. That is especially true for pain. We've been told for years that pain comes from physical conditions and abnormalities—real, hard, tangible issues with our body—but the truth is that we don't yet fully understand the science behind the pain that affects billions around the world every single day and is likely affecting you today.

To highlight just one example, let's look at low back pain. It's the most common source of pain in the United States, responsible for more than $50 billion in lost work time and worker's compensation claims each year. Many who suffer from low back pain are diagnosed with a herniated disc and told that's the cause of the pain that's robbing them of sleep, limiting their mobility, and making their daily lives feel like torture. What's surprising is that studies have found no conclusive evidence that herniated discs cause pain, especially chronic pain. Studies show that many people whose X-rays reveal a herniated disc have no pain, while others whose X-rays reveal no herniated disc (or any other abnormalities) report excruciating pain.

According to one study done by George Washington University and published in the journal *Spine,* lumbar CT scans were performed on 52 patients who had no low back pain. The neuroradiologists who reviewed the scans had no knowledge of the patients' clinical histories. They found disc abnormalities, stenosis, and other aging changes in 35.4 percent of the entire group and in 50 percent of the group over 40 years of age. The study findings suggest that these are all normal abnormalities and that they can't be conclusively linked to pain.

Let me repeat this, because I know how many people experience back pain and have been told it's because of a herniated disc: they examined dozens of CT scans that clearly indicated herniated discs, stenosis, and other abnormalities, yet none of the people had pain.

Additional statistics around pain are just as confusing. While many blame conditions like herniated discs, as well as chronic pain in general, on age, most back pain sufferers are in midlife, somewhere between 30 and 60 years old. Several studies have shown a decrease in back pain once people reach their early to mid-60s. If chronic back pain were age related, 65-year-olds would be reporting more pain, not less, than 45-year-olds do. More confounding data!

The confusion about what causes pain increases when you look at pain statistics by gender. Back pain, migraines, neck pain, facial and jaw pain, fibromyalgia, and Complex Regional Pain Syndrome (CRPS) are all more common in women than in men, but none of these conditions has been linked to gender-specific anatomy or health issues.

So where's the pain really coming from? Might our common knowledge about pain, that it's related to something being physically wrong with the body or with getting older, be just plain wrong or, at the very least, dramatically myopic?

Pain, the Brain, and Emotions

Thanks to large libraries of functional images and functional magnetic resonance imaging (fMRI) scans that show what happens in the brain when a patient experiences physical pain, we know that the brain can send signals to the body that then produce pain. We also know that the brain can take pain away. Research has also shown that emotions such as fear and anxiety can increase pain. Negative emotions may also turn short-term pain into a chronic condition.

One Dutch study on how negative emotions affect pain involved 121 women: 62 had been diagnosed with fibromyalgia, a condition that involves chronic pain, and 59 did not have the disease. Using an electrical stimulus, pain was induced in two separate circumstances: while the women recalled an emotionally neutral event and as they remembered an event that made them feel sad and/or angry. Higher levels of pain were consistently felt when the women were recalling memories that made them feel sad and/or angry.

In a separate randomized controlled trial with more than 150 patients, those who were given cognitive behavioral therapy that allowed them to express their emotions experienced less pain, fatigue, and functional disability than those who were put on a waiting list did. So how *do* emotions interact with pain in the body?

There are many different ways the brain and body can create, increase, and prolong pain. In some cases, a physical event, like picking up something heavy and hurting your back, is what initially triggers pain. In that case, nearly everyone experiences pain immediately, or very soon after the injury occurs. Immediately after, the brain's networks and neurons begin to rewire in an effort to protect you from similar future injuries—putting you on "higher alert" to avoid pain. The brain's ability to rewire is known as *neuroplasticity*. The neuroplastic changes that occur in the brain immediately after an injury vary significantly from one person to another and from one event to another.

Some experts believe that the nature and timing of the specific neuroplastic changes in the brain that happen after an injury may affect where, and for how long, you experience pain from that injury. In other words, your emotional state at the time of injury, or during the hours immediately after the injury occurs, may help to determine whether your pain will become chronic, whether it will occur in several places or just one, and so on.

First Thing First, Go See a Doctor!

If you are experiencing a new, acute pain that has no obvious explanation, be sure to consult a physician before you use tapping for pain relief. Pain is your body's way of talking to you, and medical tests may be necessary to correctly interpret what it is saying and whether a condition has developed that will worsen without medical intervention.

When Pain Becomes a Disease

There are two basic kinds of pain—acute pain and chronic pain. Acute pain is a temporary reaction of the nervous system to disease, injury, or other threats to the body, like the pain you experience immediately after falling down and hitting your knee. Chronic pain is different. It can last for anywhere from three months to years, even decades. According to pain expert Sean Mackey, M.D., Ph.D., at the Stanford University Pain Management Center, "When pain becomes persistent, it can become a disease in its own right."

Think about that for a moment. If chronic pain were a disease unto itself, then pain would be treated on its own, with little to no consideration paid to injuries or any other physical conditions, abnormalities, or ailments. That would mean you could be diagnosed with chronic low back pain, period. There would be no herniated disc or injury to blame. The pain itself would be your diagnosis. Given the close linkages between emotions and chronic pain, your doctor might then ask about your emotional state, the stressors in your life, whether you'd experienced trauma, and so on. He or she might then recommend a therapist—ideally one who uses tapping. That would be a huge shift in our thinking around pain! It would also open up new possibilities for how to treat pain.

Fortunately, there's a growing consensus that we need new ways to relieve pain. More than 100 million Americans suffer from chronic pain each year. Many are diagnosed with physical conditions and recommended for surgery. Sadly, even after surgery, many people remain in pain, or end up in greater pain because of the surgery itself. As just one example, 20 percent of patients who have a knee-replacement surgery end up with chronic pain after surgery. An even larger number are treated with costly pharmaceuticals that come with a long list of side effects and provide short-lived and, in many cases, partial pain relief. Pills and surgeries clearly aren't providing the lasting pain relief that people desperately need, so what can?

My answer? Tapping.

First developed 30 years ago by psychologist Dr. Roger Callahan, tapping has been used by tens of thousands of people to successfully relieve chronic pain. The technique brings together the best of Eastern and Western medicine, targeting both the emotional and the physical aspects of pain. It involves verbally expressing emotions, usually out loud, while tapping with your fingertips on specific meridian points on the body. After witnessing the results tapping produced in his patients, Callahan began teaching his method to other professionals. One of his students was Gary Craig, an engineer at Stanford University. Craig simplified Callahan's method and renamed it the Emotional Freedom Techniques (EFT). The EFT sequence includes nine key tapping points, which most tapping experts use today. Craig's EFT sequence, along with Dr. Patricia Carrington's Choices Method of tapping, have, as she says, made tapping "the people's method," rather than a tool available only to highly trained professionals.

Acupuncture Points Evident in Scans

Using sophisticated CT imaging, a 2013 study published in the *Journal of Electron Spectroscopy and Related Phenomena* confirmed the existence of acupuncture points. The study, which is one of several that has proven the anatomical significance of acupuncture points, demonstrated that the points have a distinct structure and a higher density of micro-vessels that are larger than those in nonacupuncture points. A separate study demonstrated that acupuncture points also have a higher partial oxygen pressure than nonacupuncture points.

Proof of the Mind–Body Connection

Even though people see a lot of amazing results from tapping, many still secretly wonder what *actually* relieved the pain. Surely it couldn't just be tapping . . . right? In fact, yes, it could. To better understand why tapping is so effective for pain relief, we can look at Candace Pert's monumental discoveries around the mind–body connection.

At the time of her research findings, Candace Pert was an unlikely candidate for changing the future of medical science. A female doctoral candidate working in the male-dominated laboratories at the National Institutes of Health (NIH) in the 1970s, it was her success in measuring the opiate receptor that provided a scientific basis for what Pert calls the bodymind. (For scientists, measurement is the gold standard. By measuring the opiate receptor, Pert was proving its existence.) As she explains in her book *Molecules of Emotion,* "Technological innovations have allowed us to examine the molecular basis of the emotions, and to begin to understand how the molecules of our emotions share intimate connections with, and are indeed inseparable from, our physiology. It is the emotions, I have come to see, that link mind and body."

Pert was a doctor of pharmacology, an author, and an internationally renowned speaker, and her discoveries have allowed us to begin to understand potential links between diseases like chronic pain and emotions. The opiate receptors Pert measured are like keyholes. They bind with very specific keys, called peptides, which, she explains, "are indeed the other half of the equation of what I call the molecules of emotion." When the opiate receptor, which floats on the surface of a cell like a lily pad on a pond, binds with its perfectly fitting peptide, that cell's behavior can change. In other words, at any given moment, a cell's behavior can shift based on which peptide "keys" are attached to its opiate receptors. "On a more global scale," Pert explains, "these minute physiological phenomena at the cellular level can translate to large changes in behavior, physical activity, even mood."

Pert's research findings have provided a scientific basis for the idea that we can heal diseases in the body by targeting emotions. As Pert shares, "It is this problem of unhealed feeling, the accumulation of bruised and broken emotions, that most people stagger under without ever saying a word, that the mainstream medical model is least effective in dealing with."

The Root Cause of Pain

John Sarno, M.D., author of *Healing Back Pain,* has seen Pert's discoveries play out on a human level throughout most of his career. In his work with thousands of patients, Sarno identified a bodymind disease he calls Tension Myositis Syndrome (TMS); *myositis* means physiologic alteration of muscle. According to Sarno, we all naturally feel negative emotions, especially anger, as a result of the

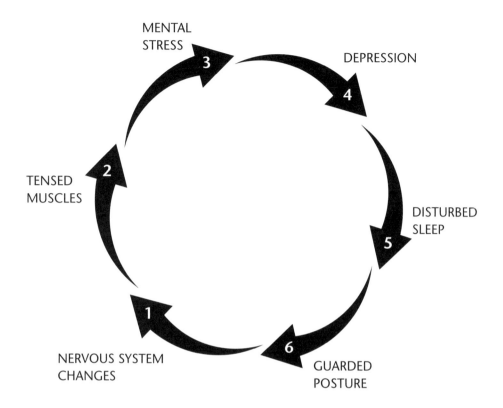

MENTAL STRESS — 3
DEPRESSION — 4
TENSED MUSCLES — 2
DISTURBED SLEEP — 5
NERVOUS SYSTEM CHANGES — 1
GUARDED POSTURE — 6

many stressors and demands of everyday life. When that anger builds over time and remains unexpressed, it can become buried in the unconscious mind. As he explains, "Accumulated anger is rage, and frightening, unconscious rage leads to the development of physical symptoms."

This process is completely normal, but it's not easily controlled by the conscious mind using conventional therapies. As Sarno explains, "Most people, if given the choice between coming to terms with difficult feelings or experiencing intense physical pain, would choose to deal with the feelings. That's logical. But the way the human emotional system is now organized dictates how it will react; at the unconscious level it is often illogical." As a result, instead of processing negative emotions like anger, we often unconsciously bury them.

Once repressed rage has reached a certain level in the unconscious mind, the brain begins to create physical symptoms, such as chronic pain, by limiting blood flow to one or several areas of the body. So let's say you went through a horrible divorce years ago. It needed to happen, and you now know you're better off as a result. You feel as if you're over it, but, in fact, while the divorce was happening, your unconscious mind buried your rage without your realizing it. That's what the unconscious mind does—it takes over without our knowledge or consent. Over time, that repressed rage limits oxygen supply to your muscles. That oxygen deprivation then leads to muscle constriction, which spreads to nearby muscles. You experience that process every time you clench your fist. First the muscles in your hand tighten, and, almost immediately after, the muscles in your lower arm tighten also. As time goes on, when your muscles remain tight and constricted, you experience pain.

Imagine if I asked you to clench your fist right now and keep it clenched. After a minute your hand might get tired. After ten minutes, maybe your hand would ache, and then pain would set in. What would happen if you kept it clenched for a whole day, month, or year? Obviously, you would experience pain, muscular degeneration, and all sorts of problems, not just in your hand but in your wrist and arm as well. Eventually your shoulder would be affected, and so on. Imagine the same thing happening in whatever part of your body is in pain. The tension builds, muscles contract, blood flow constricts, and pain follows.

According to Sarno, the only way to treat TMS is by addressing the underlying emotions that originally caused the pain: "When patients become aware of the presence of rage or unbearable feelings, these feelings can cease their struggle to become conscious. Removing that threat eliminates the need for physical distraction, and the pain stops." Sarno's work shows that we can treat physical pain by finding new ways to access the bodymind and process our emotions in a more complete way.

Open to the Possibility . . .

Even if you don't connect immediately with the concept of repressed rage (it is, after all, repressed!), begin considering if there are emotions that might be a little buried, a little stuck, a little unexplored.

Play with the idea that, perhaps, there is some tension and constriction in your muscles and your body as a result of emotional experiences that aren't fully healed and released. Just opening up your awareness to this possibility can have profound healing effects. We'll be exploring these concepts in much more detail throughout this book.

The Brain's Negativity Bias

When we're looking at how the emotions and the brain interact with pain, it's important to understand that the human brain has evolved to focus more on negative outcomes than on positive ones. For our own protection, it was built to always assume the worst—it's biased toward negativity. In his book *Hardwiring Happiness,* Rick Hanson, Ph.D., explains this concept in more detail:

> Our ancestors could make two kinds of mistakes: (1) thinking there was a tiger in the bushes when there wasn't one, and (2) thinking there was no tiger in the bushes when there actually was one. The cost of the first mistake was needless anxiety, while the cost of the second one was death. Consequently, we evolved to make the first mistake a thousand times to avoid making the second mistake even once . . . the default setting of the brain is to *over*estimate threats, *under*estimate opportunities, and *under*estimate resources both for coping with threats and for fulfilling opportunities. Then we update these beliefs with information that confirms them, while ignoring or rejecting information that doesn't. There are even regions in the amygdala specifically designed to prevent the unlearning of fear, especially from childhood experiences. As a result, we end up preoccupied by threats that are actually smaller or more manageable than we'd feared, while overlooking opportunities that are actually greater than we'd hoped for. In effect, we've got a brain that's prone to "paper tiger paranoia."

Most of us can relate to what Hanson calls "the special power of fear" because it's been hammered into our unconscious minds for millennia. Think about your daily routine. As you go about your day, if you make a movement that causes you pain, if you're like most people, you remember to avoid that movement for months afterward. If you also do something that soothes your pain or even feels good, you might not remember it as readily. That's your primitive brain at work.

In other words, because of how our brains have evolved, negative experiences routinely outweigh positive ones. The psychologist Daniel Kahnemann received the Nobel Prize in economics for showing that most people will do more to avoid loss than to benefit from an equivalent gain. In intimate relationships, we typically need at least five positive interactions to counterbalance every negative one. And for people to begin to thrive in life, they usually need positive moments to outweigh negative ones by at least a three-to-one ratio.

Again, think about yourself. Let's say you're having a good day. You're feeling good, with relatively low pain. At the very end of your day, a neighbor says something that upsets you. Do you go to bed that night thinking about what a good day you've had and how much better your body felt, or do you go to bed that night focused on what your neighbor said? Most of us will focus on what the neighbor said. That's how the brain's negativity bias works.

We can even see it in how the brain functions. The amygdala, the part of the brain that gets activated when we're under stress, and also a part of the brain involved in emotions as well as physical pain, typically gets activated more by negative experiences than by positive ones.

So I'm sure you're wondering what this has to do with tapping and pain relief. What I've seen, and what Hanson also alludes to, is that the negativity bias puts undue stress on the body. When your body is under stress or senses a threat, it secretes the hormone cortisol, which is also referred to as the "stress hormone." The threat that you're experiencing can be physical, like getting out of the way of an oncoming car, or emotional, such as feeling anxious, angry, or afraid. When you experience ongoing stress for a long period of time, your body releases excessive amounts of cortisol, which may make you more susceptible to pain and less likely to heal from injury or experience pain relief.

When you're feeling more positive, the body is in a more relaxed state, and cortisol levels naturally go down. The body is then better able to support healing in the body, as well as pain relief.

Tapping Into the Body's Natural Painkillers

Up to this point, we've looked at how the body, emotions, and stress interact to create pain. So how does tapping figure into the science of pain and, more important, pain relief and the bodymind?

While we don't have all the answers about why tapping works so well for pain relief, there's a growing body of research on the topic. In a double-blind study conducted by Dawson Church, Ph.D., tapping was shown to produce, on average, a 24 percent drop in cortisol after just one hour of tapping. During that same hour of talk therapy without tapping, participants showed a much smaller drop in cortisol levels.

That drop in cortisol may be partially responsible for the pain relief tapping provides, and there are numerous studies that show how effective tapping is for pain relief. One randomized control study of patients suffering from tension headaches at the Red Cross Hospital in Athens showed a 50+ percent decrease in the intensity and frequency of headaches after tapping. A different study examined 216 health-care workers, who experienced a 68 percent drop in physical pain after a one-day tapping workshop. Separate studies involving veterans as well as fibromyalgia sufferers have also shown significant decreases in physical pain after tapping.

Research has shown that acupuncture, and potentially acupressure as well, provides pain relief by increasing endorphin levels in the body. Since tapping engages acupressure points while also lowering cortisol, it's likely that tapping, like acupuncture, allows the body to release the endorphins that then relieve pain.

Chronic Pain in Phantom Limbs

Studies have repeatedly shown that a significant percentage of people who lose limbs experience chronic pain in those missing limbs. In one study published by the NIH, almost 80 percent of amputees reported suffering from chronic pain in their missing limbs. And for many of them, the pain was severe.

Interestingly, tapping has proven to be extraordinarily successful with phantom-limb pain. Carey Mann, an EFT practitioner based in London, who's also a friend of mine, has worked with clients who suffer from phantom-limb pain. Ben Mcbean is one of those clients. A soldier who lost his right leg and left arm in 2008 after stepping on a land mine in Afghanistan, he suffered from phantom-limb pain for five years. Throughout that time, his pain had ranged from moderate to severe in intensity.

During Carey's session with Ben, she tapped through the points on his body while having him remember the trauma he'd experienced the day of the explosion. As he began to feel the heat sensations he'd felt during and right after the explosion, as well as several challenging emotions, Carey had Ben distance himself from his memories. Rather than reliving it, she had him go back to that day as his current and older self to reassure his younger self that he was going to be okay. As he did that, he hit several points during his memories that caused his fear and anxiety to spike. Each time that happened, Carey had him pause and tap through that piece of his memory until it was cleared. (These are all tapping techniques we'll cover in more detail throughout this book, so you'll have plenty of time to experience them for yourself.)

By the end of the session, Ben's phantom-limb pain had decreased a great deal. In fact, it felt less like pain and more like buzzing. Within the three weeks that followed their tapping session, Ben's pain disappeared completely. For the first time since losing his limbs, he was able to begin living his life without pain and without focusing so much of his time and energy on his phantom limbs.

You can watch Carey's session with Ben Mcbean on her YouTube channel at: www.youtube.com/user/CareyMannTV.

In other cases, such as someone who has debilitating back pain but has no herniated discs or other abnormalities, the brain may be creating very real physical pain in the body without an obvious physical trigger. Fortunately, a growing amount of research is giving us a better understanding of what pain is and how to relieve it.

The incredible results that tapping has in alleviating chronic pain may be explained, at least in part, by its ability to access what are called meridian channels. While knowledge of these channels dates back to ancient Chinese medicine, it wasn't until the 1960s that these threadlike microscopic anatomical structures were first seen on stereomicroscope and electron microscope images. These scans showed tubular structures measuring 30 to 100 micrometers wide running up and down the body. Described in a published paper by a North Korean researcher named Kim Bonghan, they are also referred to as "Bonghan channels." As a reference point, one red blood cell is 6 to 8 micrometers wide, so these structures are tiny!

You can think of meridian channels as a fiber-optic network in the body. They carry a large amount of information, often electrical and often beyond what the nervous system or chemical systems of the body can carry. By accessing these channels while processing emotions and thoughts as well as physical conditions like pain, some suggest that tapping is able to get to the root cause of chronic pain more quickly than other approaches can.

Because tapping sends calming, relaxing signals directly to the amygdala, it may also help us to override the brain's negativity bias more rapidly. By using tapping to neutralize what it thought were threats to its survival, we may be able to reprogram the brain to support more positive experiences, such as pain relief, pleasure, and relaxation.

So let's look at just one example now of how powerful tapping can be.

Chronic Pain and Infection . . . Gone!

"It was awful," Cathy Shipley said of the three and a half years she spent suffering from constant tooth pain and infection, which, many times, was excruciating. Since undergoing major dental work, which included bone grafts and much more, Cathy had spent years living on antibiotics and pain medicine. As the years and the pain piled on, she began to realize that conventional medicine simply didn't seem able to heal her pain. Desperate to get her life back, she began researching alternative options and eventually took a flight to attend a conference where I was one of a number of teachers.

After the lunch break on the first day of the event, she felt discouraged, worried that her pain would never go away, but she sat back down in her seat anyway to listen to the next presenter, who happened to be me. Having never heard of tapping or of me, she raised her hand when I asked for volunteers who were in physical pain and who were willing to share their stories with me onstage and try tapping.

When she came up onstage, we began by doing some tapping on her anxiety around being onstage and trying this "weird tapping thing." Then I asked her what can often be a powerful question when it comes to pain: "What was happening in your life when the tooth pain began?"

She paused for a moment, then gasped as she realized that around the same time her tooth pain started, her mom had passed away during a family trip to Las Vegas. It was clear that Cathy hadn't made the connection between her tooth pain and her mom's death until that moment onstage, in front of 3,000 people. We did some tapping around her memories of her mom's passing, as well as her grief and other emotions related to the event. By the end of our 25 or so minutes tapping together, Cathy's pain was almost entirely gone. For the first time in three and a half years, Cathy was, much to her surprise and the delight of the audience, nearly pain-free.

Excited by her progress, I kept in touch with Cathy. Some time into our correspondence, she told me that her pain had actually begun to return a few days after the event. Scared that her results wouldn't last, she immediately read my first book, *The Tapping Solution: A Revolutionary System for Stress-Free Living,* which I had given her after we'd tapped together onstage. Through reading that book, she learned how to tap on her own. As soon as she began tapping again, going even deeper on the emotional issues than we'd had a chance to do onstage, her pain went away. This time, however, it disappeared completely, never to return!

Here's an e-mail she sent me several months later explaining everything she'd been through:

Hi Nick!

It started when I broke a tooth on a piece of candy. To fix that tooth they wanted to make a bridge using a healthy tooth, which is the tooth that wouldn't heal. I then changed dentists. From there they used more teeth as you can see in the X-rays. The dentist I have now did everything to help it heal. Here's the breakdown:

- One broken tooth.
- Then bridge using one additional tooth . . . healthy tooth went bad.
- Changed dentist.
- Did a root canal on healthy tooth that went bad.
- Mom died.
- Root canal went bad.
- Tooth next to it went bad (no idea why).
- Extracted teeth.
- Put in implants.
- Implants went bad (I got so discouraged at this point).
- Did bone graft.
- Didn't work.

- Did extensive bone graft (heavily sedated for this one). With both bone grafts, they took out the implants, rolled them in antibiotics, and put them back in! UGH! Took out bone and put in new bone.

- Second bone graft became infected.

- Antibiotics for 6 to 8 weeks at a time (I was on antibiotics . . . more on than off, for almost three years).

- Went to DC . . . TAPPED WITH YOU. Pain went away. YAY!

- Got home, three days later started hurting again, finished your book, tapped more on the feelings of loss and it healed. Go figure!

- ALL of the above included X-rays with each visit and sometimes just went in for X-rays because it hurt due to infection.

I have been tapping for almost eight months, and I'm pain-free, and infection-free, not to mention finally antibiotic-free! I will tell you this: every day I say a prayer for you, for your love and compassion to help those who need help to pinpoint a reason for their pain. When you are so close, you often don't see it, which is why you are such a blessing. I truly believe my mom, my angels (and yours), God, and probably others lined up the things as they did for me to be onstage. You are a godsend. I will tell my grandchildren about you!

As exciting as Cathy's pain relief is, perhaps the most amazing part of her story is about her tooth infection, which had been noticeably inflamed since her dental surgery three and a half years previously. After using tapping to get rid of her pain, Cathy went back to her doctor and got X-rays to check on the infection. She and the doctor were amazed to see that just two weeks after doing her first round of tapping, Cathy's infection was completely gone. She was so excited that she sent me her X-rays from before and after tapping. Here they are:

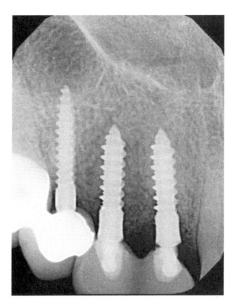

X-ray before tapping: The dark areas in the image above,
clearly show Cathy's chronic tooth infection

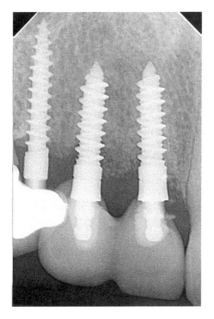

X-ray after tapping.

In contrast with the first X-ray picture, the areas that were previously dark are now light, indicating that the infection has healed, as evidenced by her pain disappearing.

A couple of weeks after getting those X-rays, Cathy attended a three-day tapping for pain relief event I hosted and got onstage to share her journey with the audience. "For the first time in three and a half years," she explained, "I can smile big without feeling excruciating pain. It makes me so happy."

By clearing the emotions that had been in some way taking a toll on her body since her mom's death, Cathy's body had finally been able to do what conventional medicine had been unable to do—heal her chronic tooth pain and infection. It's a powerful reminder of how closely connected our emotions are to the body.

Tapping Can Work for Anyone

One of the things I love about tapping is that it can be used by anyone, in any place, at any time. It works on people of all ages, with all kinds of diagnoses and health issues. As you'll see next, there is no one way to use tapping for pain relief. While this book lays out a process that's meant to guide you, I invite you to use it to create your own personal journey to a pain-free life. Whether you choose to use tapping on your own or work with an EFT professional, the possibilities for what tapping can do to relieve your pain and help you live a healthier, more vibrant life are nearly endless.

So now that we've explored some of the science behind it, you're probably ready to start tapping!

CHAPTER 2

RAPID PAIN RELIEF RIGHT NOW

It was the second morning of a three-day pain-relief event I was conducting in Stamford, Connecticut, in the fall of 2013. Walking onstage, I was glad to see more smiling faces in the audience than I had the previous morning—it's always a good sign that we're moving in the right direction when it comes to pain relief. When I began the morning by asking if anyone had experienced a shift overnight, several hands shot up. Nancy was the first to come up onstage to share her story.

Holding the mic, she explained that she'd been suffering from chronic headaches, which were usually accompanied by neck discomfort and nausea, for 12 years. Prior to attending the event, she'd had a headache every day and night for three weeks straight. During the previous day's sessions, we'd done a lot of tapping, but when the final session of the day had ended, much to her dismay, her headache was still raging.

Upon returning to her room at the end of the day, however, Nancy had done more tapping with a friend who was also attending the event. They took turns and tapped on issues that had come up while watching people onstage throughout the day. As Nancy tapped while voicing her own reactions to the day, she had a huge breakthrough around her headaches. Excited about her breakthrough but still in pain, she went to sleep. When she woke up in the morning, she was amazed that her headache, as well as her neck discomfort and nausea, were completely gone. Within 24 hours' time, she'd been able to resolve 12 years of nearly constant pain. Wow!

The goal of any tapping, whether it's a simple five minutes or an extended three-day event, is to have a shift that tells us we're moving in the right direction. Even the pain decreasing a tiny amount in intensity means that a shift is happening, so acknowledge that as positive progress. This is one of the ways we can begin to overcome the brain's negativity bias—by pausing and taking in every positive shift and experience, no matter how big or small. You should also tune in to any emotional shift—no matter the scale. Tune in to insights and feelings as you begin this journey toward complete and lasting pain relief. This is what will lead to experiencing amazing results like Nancy's.

Oftentimes the best place to start—and get the most rapid pain relief—is by tapping through the points while focusing on the pain itself. So let's learn how to tap by focusing our attention here.

Direct Tapping on the Pain

One of the great things about tapping is how easy it is to get started. Below, we'll go over each step in detail.

Step 1: Focus on Your Pain

Before tapping on your pain, you first need to focus your attention on it. This step may feel uncomfortable, since you may have spent weeks, months, or years trying to train yourself *not* to focus on your pain. To get results, however, I need you to put that effort aside and place your full attention on your pain, if only for a few minutes while we do this process. Begin by getting your journal. If you have pain in multiple places, start with the one that's most noticeable. Then ask yourself the following: *If my pain were a color, what color would it be? Does it have a texture and/or shape? A sound? Does it feel hot? Is it dull or sharp? Does it radiate or stay still? Does it look like a wave? A hammer? A razor-sharp pin?* Write your answers in your journal, and try to be as specific as possible about how it looks and feels to you. We're trying to get a full physical sensation of the pain, not only to tap on it but to be able to better notice as it shifts.

Step 2: Measure the Intensity of Your Pain

Now that you've gotten a clearer sense of your pain, I want you to give your pain a number on a 0-to-10 scale. This is called the SUDS, or Subjective Units of Distress Scale. When you focus on the pain you're feeling right now, how intense does it feel at this moment? A 10 would be the most pain you can imagine; a 0 would mean you don't feel any pain at all. Don't worry about getting the SUDS level exact or "right"—just follow your gut instinct. If your low back is in agony right now and the pain is impossible to ignore, you might rate it an 8 or a 9. If you're in pain, but not as much as you generally feel when you lie down on your back, for example, you might rate it a 6. To see a significant shift, start with pain you can rate at 5 or higher. In your journal, write down the SUDS number for the pain you will be addressing.

Step 3: Craft Your Setup Statement

With your SUDS level in mind, your next step is to craft what's called the "setup statement." This statement focuses on the energy and nature of your pain. Once you know your setup statement, you can start tapping.

The basic setup statement might go like this:

Even though I <describe your pain>,
I deeply and completely love and accept myself.

So, for example, you might say, "Even though I have this hot, sharp, stabbing pain in my lower back, I deeply and completely love and accept myself."

Or, "Even though I have this dull, throbbing pain in my jaw, I deeply and completely accept myself."

Your setup statement should resonate with what you're experiencing when you begin tapping. The goal is not to say magic words as if they're the formula that unlocks the door to pain relief. You want to say words that have *meaning* to you, so if the basic setup statement doesn't ring true or feel powerful, change it.

Here are a few (of many!) variations on the basic setup statement that you can use and change to fit your experience:

Even though I <describe your pain>, I completely love, accept, and forgive myself and anyone else.

Even though I <describe your pain>, I choose to forgive myself now.

Even though I <describe your pain>, I accept and forgive myself.

Even though I <describe your pain>, I allow myself to be the way I am.

Even though I <describe your pain>, I'm willing to let go.

Even though I <describe your pain>, I'm willing to hold a new perspective.

Even though I <describe your pain>, it's over and I'm safe now.

Even though I <describe your pain>, I choose to release this pain now.

The Choices Method

EFT expert Dr. Patricia Carrington's Choices Method is another great option for creating your setup statement. Using her method, you counter what you're feeling and add "and I choose . . ." at the end. For example, if you're feeling frustrated, you could use the setup statement "Even though I'm feeling frustrated with this pain, I choose to feel calm and patient and release this pain now."

Step 4: Choose a Reminder Phrase

The reminder phrase is short—just a few words that describe your pain. After you say your setup statement three times while tapping on the karate chop point (see page 23), you will speak your reminder phrase out loud at each of the eight points in the tapping sequence (see page 23). For example, if your setup statement has to do with the pain in your lower back, you might tap through each point in the sequence saying, "This pain in my lower back . . . this pain in my lower back . . . this pain in my lower back . . ."

You're repeating the reminder phrase out loud to remind yourself of the issue at each point. This reminder phrase serves to keep your focus on the pain so you don't get distracted. It also acts as a barometer, helping you determine along the way how the pain feels.

Once you get used to tapping, you can change your reminder phrase as you tap through each point. For example, you might say, "All this pain in my lower back . . . this stabbing pain in my lower back . . . this hot, stabbing pain . . ." I will offer this kind of evolving reminder phrase in the tapping scripts throughout the book. But to start with, feel free to keep it simple and say the same statement at each point.

Step 5: Tap Through the Points

Once you have created your setup statement and your reminder phrase, you're ready to start tapping. You'll start by saying your setup statement three times, all the while tapping on the karate chop point. You can tap with whichever hand feels most comfortable to you. Tap at a pace and force that feel right; you can't get it wrong!

After you've said the setup statement three times, you'll move on to tapping through the eight points in the tapping sequence while saying the reminder phrase. These points are:

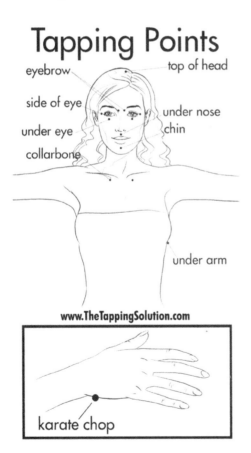

1. Eyebrow
2. Side of eye
3. Under eye
4. Under nose
5. Chin
6. Collarbone
7. Under arm
8. Top of head

You can tap with either hand, on whichever side of the body feels best to you, because the same meridian channels run down both sides of the body. You can even tap both sides of the body at once if you'd like (it's not necessary, however, as you'll hit the same meridian lines, regardless of which side you tap). Tap five to seven times at each stop as you work through the sequence. This doesn't have to be an exact count. If it feels right to tap 20 times—or 100—on one point, then do it! The idea is simply to spend enough time at that point to speak your reminder phrase and let it sink in. Don't worry about getting it perfect; just do your best and have the experience.

Step 6: Check In

You've now completed a round of tapping! First things first: Take a deep breath. Feel your body and notice what's happening. Did your pain shift? How does it feel on the 0-to-10 scale now? If your pain went from an 8 to a 7, that's huge! It means that tapping is beginning to relieve your pain. It means a shift happened in just a matter of minutes, so keep tapping. If there's no change, that's fine, too. It's common for people to need more than one round of tapping to experience relief, especially as they are becoming familiar with the process.

You may notice yourself yawning, sighing, burping, or experiencing other physical side effects during or after tapping. These are all ways that your body is moving and releasing energy, relaxing, and letting go. When you tap, make a point of noticing all these ways that your body is responding.

Also, as you check in with yourself to see if your pain has changed, ask yourself what thoughts or emotions came up while tapping. It may be hard in the beginning if you're focused on learning the points and getting the process right, but these will be important clues later in the process as we begin exploring the deeper cause of your pain.

Switching from the "Negative" to the "Positive"

As you'll notice in the tapping scripts throughout the book, each one begins with the "negative," a statement that includes the physical pain itself, as well as stress and other challenging emotions and beliefs. Most of the time, I'll end with at least one "positive" round of tapping, which presents a new way of moving forward. As a general rule, it's best to get the intensity of the "negative" down to a 5 out of 10 before moving on to the "positive," and then to keep tapping on the positive until the negative emotional charge has decreased to a 3 or lower.

As you tap, remember to tune in to any shifts you experience in your pain, small or large. Tune in to how your body and your emotional state are shifting. Tune in to new insights and feelings as you begin this journey toward complete and lasting pain relief.

Chasing the Pain: One thing you may notice as you go through the tapping process is that your pain shifts. It may move to a new location, go from sharp to dull, begin to tingle, radiate, or change character in some other way. Occasionally, your pain may even increase when you first begin tapping. Remember that these are all signs that tapping is impacting your pain. That's good! When you experience any kind of shift in your pain, you can then tap on the new pain you're feeling, or the new place on your body where you're feeling pain, and so on. This is what's called "chasing the pain."

Tapping Tip: Stick with Me . . .

If you find yourself tapping but not noticing any changes yet, that's okay, too. This is the beginning of a longer process that has had results for tens of thousands of people who suffer from chronic pain. Keep tapping, and if you feel frustrated or scared that this process won't work for you, make sure to include those emotions in your tapping.

To most people, tapping seems strange at first. It takes a little effort to memorize the points and understand the process. But stick with me through the process and take the time to really learn the basic steps. The investment you make now will make all the difference.

Step 7: Test Your Progress

Once your pain has decreased or even shifted to a new location, it's time to test your results. Often we do this by doing something like making a movement that may typically cause you pain. For example, if you usually feel pain in your neck when you move in a certain way, then make that movement after you tap. You might find that the pain, which would usually be unbearable when you moved in that way, is now less intense than it usually is. In that case, tap a few more rounds using the same language and see if you can clear the pain altogether.

Or you might find that, as you made that movement, you felt pain in your shoulder instead of your neck. That's great! That's an indication that your pain is responding to tapping. In that case, you can move on and tap on the pain in your shoulder you feel when you make that specific movement. This is another example of "chasing the pain."

Tapping Process: Quick Reference Guide

Now that we've been through the tapping process in detail, here's a quick step-by-step guide for reference:

1. To start, close your eyes and take three deep breaths. Feel yourself grounded in your body and focused on the present moment. Feel your feet firmly planted on the ground, rooted to the earth. We want to give this process and your body all the attention it deserves, so take a few moments to become present.

2. Focus on your pain (or whatever issue is bothering you most) and devise a setup statement (see page 21). Write down in your journal what kind of pain you're feeling (sharp, dull, hot, cold, etc.) and where it is located.

3. Rate the intensity of your pain on the 0-to-10 SUDS (see page 21), with 10 being the most excruciating pain you can imagine. Note this number in your journal.

4. Craft a setup statement (see page 21).

---

5. Tap on the karate chop point (see page 23) while repeating your setup statement three times.

6. Tap through the eight points in the EFT sequence (see page 23) while saying your reminder phrase out loud. Tap five to seven times at each point, but don't worry about counting or doing it perfectly; it's a forgiving process.

7. Once you have finished tapping the points in the sequence, take a deep breath, and check in. Again rate the intensity of your pain using the 0-to-10 scales to check your progress.

8. Test your progress by doing the movement that caused pain, or focusing on the memory or emotion that increased your pain.

9. Continue tapping as necessary to get the relief you desire.

10. In your journal, write down the shifts you experience in your pain, and note any changes in pain intensity as well. Remember, shifts in your pain mean progress!

Tracking Your Progress

Throughout this process, as you know already, I'll be asking you to record your experience in a journal dedicated exclusively to your tapping for pain relief. Write down what you're experiencing physically and emotionally at the beginning and end (and in the middle, when needed) of each tapping experience. Keeping a brief history will help to guide you as you get deeper into this journey.

Tapping Targets

So far, we've focused our tapping on the physical sensation of pain. That's often a great and simple starting point for rapid pain relief. Throughout this book, however, we'll explore several deeper layers to find the original cause of your pain, which in many cases is the key to achieving complete and lasting pain relief. Whatever issue is being tapped on in any given round is called the "target." As you tap, different layers or aspects of that target will arise. Often you start with one target and then find something else underneath it—a layer! For example, your initial target might be the pain you feel in your foot. As you tap on that pain, it may shift—and at the same time, you may realize that you feel frustrated that your pain won't seem to go away.

Then, as you tap through that frustration, you may remember your doctor telling you there was nothing more he or she could do, and how much rage and fear you felt at that moment. And so it continues, until you work through all the layers of your foot pain. Working through these layers might seem tedious at first, but chronic pain is often multilayered and closely linked to emotions that aren't obvious. Unless we address every layer or aspect of your pain, we can't hope to relieve it fully. And beyond relieving the pain fully, we get the added benefit of relieving the emotional component! Yes, a pill might be able to relieve the pain in your body (for a short while, until you have to take another), but does it do anything to relieve the anger, frustration, sadness, and other emotions that come with the pain? Of course not. We're focusing on tapping for pain relief in this book, but we're really getting so many more benefits as we go deeper, in experiencing emotional relief and in truly seeing our whole lives transform.

There are four most common types of targets we will work with throughout this book: *symptoms/side effects, emotions, events,* and *limiting beliefs.*

In order to help you identify these targets in your mind, I'd like to introduce you to a great visual called the tapping tree, a concept that was created by my friend and EFT expert Lindsay Kenny. This creative visual shows each target category and how it affects particular targets.

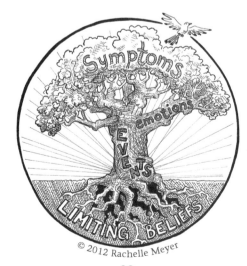

© 2012 Rachelle Meyer

The Tapping Tree: Identify Your Targets

Symptoms/Side Effects (The Leaves): This is your physical pain. If you have pain in more than one place, you may need to consider each pain point a separate symptom.

Emotions (The Branches): Shame, guilt, remorse, rejection, anger, resentment, sadness, depression, powerlessness, fear, anxiety, stress, and so on.

Events (The Trunk): Doctor visits, hospital stays, injuries, divorce, detached parents, being bullied, abandonment/betrayal, abuse in any form, overdiscipline/ criticism, physical punishment, family fighting/shouting, feeling unsupported or unloved, living with an alcoholic parent or child, and so on.

Limiting Beliefs (The Roots): "My pain will never go away," "My body is broken," "There's nothing I can do; I was diagnosed with a degenerative disease/condition," "I don't deserve to be pain-free," "Nothing more can be done for my pain; the doctors told me so," and so on.

Throughout the rest of the book, we'll skip around to various points in the tapping tree—tapping on the symptom (pain), emotions, traumatic events, and underlying beliefs alike. You may find that when you tap on one part of the tree, such as your anger at your doctor, another part of the tree, such as your pain, goes away or shifts in some way. The tree isn't necessarily a top-down or bottom-up system, since all parts feed each other and can be interrelated, but it's a useful visual to recognize the different aspects of an issue and see that it's often about much more than just the pain.

Symptoms and Side Effects (The Leaves)

We've already done some tapping on your pain, which is your symptom or "leaf." When symptom tapping doesn't get the job done, you'll know you need to go further down the tapping tree to identify a deeper target that will yield the pain relief you're looking for. A good first step is to look at your emotional state.

Emotions (The Branches)

When Cathy Shipley, the woman we met who had chronic tooth pain and infection, came up onstage to work with me, she was surprised to discover a link between her pain and her emotions around her mom's death. When she used tapping to process those emotions, she began to experience the pain relief she'd spent years searching for.

Often there are multiple emotions behind the pain. What starts as anger at a diagnosis might move into sadness, then into deep grief about all the time spent suffering. Remember, also, you can always start by tapping on emotions directly; if what's most pressing is an emotion, then that's where you should start, even if the emotion doesn't seem to be related to your pain.

Sometimes it's easy to get stuck on the emotions we're most familiar with. For example, many of us end up tapping on feelings of anger and sadness, which are easy to recognize. But accessing a broader emotional vocabulary can help bring more specificity to tapping. Here are some key emotions many of us experience. Use this list to further connect with what's going on for you.

Alienation	Envy	Hysteria
Ambivalence	Fear	Insecurity
Anger	Frustration	Loathing
Anxiety	Fury	Loneliness
Bitterness	Grief	Paranoia
Boredom	Grouchiness	Pity
Contempt	Guilt	Rage
Depression	Hatred	Regret
Despair	Homesickness	Remorse
Disgust	Horror	Resentment
Distress	Hostility	Shame
Doubt	Humiliation	Suffering
Dread	Hunger	Worry
Embarrassment		

Past Events (The Trunk)

Another common category of tapping target is past events. Chronic pain can be linked to past events that stay with us emotionally and energetically. Cathy's mom's death is a perfect example of an event that hadn't been processed on an emotional level and later contributed to her chronic pain and infection.

Tapping Tip: The Movie Technique

The Movie Technique was borrowed by EFT founder Gary Craig from another healing modality—neurolinguistic programming (NLP)—as a way to address specific events while not getting caught up in more global issues. This method consists of imagining what happened to you as a movie you are narrating. This helps keep you focused on one specific event. A movie has a beginning and an end. There are central characters who do and say specific things, and there is a usually a crescendo, or peak moment. Use the movie technique to work through a specific memory or event from your past that still holds an energetic charge.

One of the really great things about this technique is that at no point in this movie is it necessary for you to tell or say the details out loud: *you can do the whole thing in your head while tapping along.* The critical part is that the details of the movie engage all five senses. Focus on the sights, sounds, emotions, physical feelings, and what the characters are thinking and, if appropriate, smelling or tasting. The following questions will help you to set the stage for your movie.

How long will the movie last? You want to make sure it is short—three minutes or less. Often the key traumatic event in the movie takes only seconds. If there are several peaks or traumatic moments in the movie, break the experience down into as many three-minute movies as necessary.

What will the title be? Create a name specific to that movie segment.

Now that you have a specific event that has been turned into a short movie with a title, run the film in your mind. On a scale of 0 to 10, evaluate the intensity of the emotions you experience as you imagine the scene. If it feels unsafe to feel the event or emotion too deeply, you can also *guess* what your intensity would be were you to vividly imagine it.

Next, do several rounds of tapping while running the movie in your mind.

Check back on the intensity. Typically it will have come down by several points.

Then run the movie in your mind again. This time, start from a point that has no intensity or a very low intensity—and *stop and begin tapping whenever you feel the intensity arise.* This is very important! Most of us have lived with trauma for so long that we don't even notice how we push ourselves through the story, regardless of how it feels. Not anymore! With EFT, when we recognize these moments of intensity, it provides us with the perfect opportunity for tapping.

Run through the movie in your mind again, beginning to end, stopping to tap on any intense aspects as they come up. Continue until you can play the entire movie without any charge arising.

Finally, run the movie one more time. Exaggerate the sights, sounds, and colors. Really *try* to get upset about it. If you find some intensity coming back up, stop and tap again!

Note: It can be helpful to speak the events of your movie out loud, narrating it as if you were telling the story to a friend. Be sure you stop at any point that is upsetting—even just a little bit—and tap again until you are at a 0. Then continue the narration of the movie where you left off. If it feels more comfortable for you, you can tap in silence, just seeing the movie in your mind, or you can use language to describe what you see and what you feel. It's up to you!

Limiting Beliefs (The Roots)

Limiting beliefs are false beliefs about ourselves or the world, incorrect conclusions we draw based on events or experiences. For example, you may believe that your pain won't go away because your doctor said there was nothing more that he or she could do. Any idea that cuts off the possibility of pain relief, health, and wellness is a limiting belief.

Sometimes, we have beliefs from childhood that create challenging emotions that later surface in the form of pain. We get those beliefs from our parents, teachers, and peers during our early years, and they color everything in our lives from there. Beliefs like "I can't do anything right" or "I'm not good enough" are going to have profound implications on everything we do. They will change how we behave, what we say, what we pursue, and much more. Over time, they can also generate unconscious emotions that then appear as pain.

Limiting beliefs often feel like "the truth," which can make them hard to identify at first. Oftentimes, tapping on traumatic events and emotions, especially ones from childhood, can help us to reveal our limiting beliefs.

Create Your Own Tapping Tree

The Tapping Tree is a fantastic visual representation that shows how your pain might be connected to an emotion, event, or belief—how the "leaf" relates to the "branch," "trunk," or "roots." These connections and insights are vital for you to get the best pain-relief results with tapping. As I've mentioned already and will continue to mention, it's crucial that you get specific when you tap, to really home in on what's happening, and the best way to arrive at that specificity is to dig deeper to find the root cause of your pain.

To begin that process, take a few minutes now to create your own Tapping Tree. You can print out a blank copy of this drawing by visiting thetappingsolution.com/tree, or simply sketch your own on a piece of paper or in your journal. It doesn't have to be pretty, just be sure to leave plenty of space. Most of us have more stuff going on than this tree shows!

- **The Leaves—Symptoms and Side Effects:** Where do you currently feel pain? What have you been diagnosed with? Fill in all these visible, tangible issues as the leaves. For example, you might write in symptoms such as "low back pain" and "degenerative spinal condition." You can also write other side effects of the pain, such as "low energy," "can't work," and so forth.

- **The Branches—Emotions:** What emotions do you feel on a regular basis? When you feel pain, what emotions do you feel? Think back over the past day and write in any of the negative emotions you have experienced. Refer to the emotion list on page 30 if you get stuck.

- **The Trunk—Events:** Are there any events that come to mind when you think about your pain? Are there certain times of day when you feel the most pain? Does your pain get worse or change in some way when you go to work, try to exercise, or interact with a certain person? What was going on in your life when your pain started or first became chronic? In upcoming chapters, we'll dive deeper into how the past is affecting you, so don't worry about finding every single event for now. Just note the ones that seem most obvious and important.

- **The Roots—Limiting Beliefs:** What beliefs do you have about your pain? About your body? About living a pain-free life? About your health? About your ability to heal? Don't worry if you struggle coming up with these now, because they often require deeper exploration. Remember, until we recognize them as such, limiting beliefs simply feel like the truth. Some good questions to ask yourself to start bringing up some of those beliefs are:

  - What do I believe to be true about my pain?
  - What do I believe to be true about my body?
  - What do I believe to be true about my diagnosis (if relevant)?
  - What do I believe to be true about my future?

Again, we'll explore each of these in detail throughout the book. For now, just write what comes to mind.

When you're done, step back and take a look at your tree. This is a brief summary of your current challenges around pain. You'll likely discover other issues as you begin tapping, but hopefully this tree serves two purposes. First, it will help you see some of what seemingly unrelated issues may be affecting your pain. Second, it will show you how to approach tapping for the best results. These emotions, symptoms, events, and limiting beliefs are what we will be addressing throughout the book. We'll be clearing them once and for all, in order to make way for real and lasting pain relief.

If the Pain Persists, Keep Tapping!

One of the amazing benefits of EFT is how quickly it can produce real, long-lasting pain relief, regardless of the diagnosis, condition, duration, or severity of the pain, but as we've seen, the process is often different from one person to another. Sometimes people tap on the pain itself, or immediately home in on the cause of their pain, and get complete pain relief really quickly. We call these one-minute wonders, and they often happen when you least expect them. But no matter how frequently they occur, they're not the norm. We all have deep-seated emotional patterns that can be hard to break, and our brains are hardwired to resist change of all kinds. That hardwired resistance may even be the whole reason you have chronic pain! Your brain may be so adept at avoiding the emotions it doesn't want to face that it instructed your body to create chronic pain so you don't notice those emotions. For many people with chronic pain, it's the ongoing commitment to tapping that yields the relief they're seeking.

For especially deep-seated emotions—the thickest, gnarliest emotions—your tapping journey may also occasionally take unexpected turns. Remember, if the thing you're trying to clear, which could be your pain or an underlying emotion, initially gets worse while tapping, you know you are on the right path. When you start opening up to the deeper causes of your pain, a lot of repressed material can start to surface. Try not to get discouraged; it's your body's way of telling you exactly how much emotional energy it's been storing around a particular issue. I've worked with clients who start crying as soon as they tap, even without looking at emotional issues, because their bodies begin to experience and release buried emotions. If you keep tapping, you keep clearing away what's contributing to your pain. The results you can achieve in those cases, whether in minutes, hours, or weeks, are truly life changing.

When Should You Tap?

I recommend tapping whenever you feel pain, discomfort, stress, or any kind of emotional distress. There's no wrong time to tap, and it's impossible to tap too much. Some people find it helpful to make a habit of always tapping at a certain time of day, like first thing in the morning, especially if that's when you're most aware of your pain. You can also tap when you're in a challenging situation, like when you're having a difficult conversation with someone on the phone. Whenever you need relief of any kind, just start tapping!

Pain Relief Really *Is* Possible

I know that, in the beginning, tapping can seem a little confusing and strange, but once you experience some relief, be it a small shift or a huge decrease in your pain, you'll know that this is worth implementing in your life. Love yourself enough to take at least 15 minutes to experience tapping right now.

Just imagine what your life might look like on the other side of your pain, when your time and energy are no longer consumed by suffering. What might it be like to wake up pain-free every morning? What could you create, accomplish, or contribute if pain wasn't controlling your every moment? The journey begins right now. Are you ready? Let's get started!

(If you'd like further instructions highlighting the points and process of tapping, you can see a video at: thetappingsolution.com/tappingvideo.)

Audio Bonus: Tapping on the Pain Itself

I recognize that sometimes it can be hard to do the tapping on your own, so throughout the book, at relevant points, I'll be providing access to a free "tapping meditation" where I guide you through 10 to 15 minutes of tapping. I highly encourage you to take advantage of this resource. It's completely free, and you can download it to an iPod or your phone and listen at any time.

The first meditation takes you through the process of tapping on the pain itself, guiding you through it step by step. You can listen and download it for free here: thetappingsolution.com/painbookresources.

While these tapping meditations are an added bonus, I do believe they're an integral part of the book and this process, so please use them along the way. They can be just what you need to get started on the tapping and to make your experience more powerful and effective.

CHAPTER 3

RELEASING CHRONIC STRESS AND TENSION

"I'm in pain. It hurts. And it feels like my life is falling apart." Simple, direct, heartbreaking, and something I hear from clients often. They're in constant pain; many are trying to cope with limited mobility, poor sleep, and more while managing everyday stressors like relationships, work, and money. It's a lot to deal with every day, and it's no surprise that, in addition to their physical pain, most people who deal with chronic pain are seriously stressed out.

That stress itself, unfortunately, becomes part of a vicious cycle, releasing high levels of cortisol into your system and increasing emotions like anxiety and fear, which are universally recognized to amplify pain. Once stress becomes chronic, it keeps your body on high alert—an alarm that never goes off. Your muscles remain tense, and your nervous system is under constant duress, both of which can amplify your pain. The stress you feel can also prevent you from connecting to your body, which, as we'll see, is an important part of the pain-relief process.

Beginning in this chapter and continuing throughout the rest of the book, I'm going to be asking you to take a closer look at your body, at what you're experiencing, both physically and emotionally. I know that can be challenging when you want the exact opposite—to not feel your body—to find a way to turn it off! You'd much rather disconnect from your body because it's causing you so much pain. But you'll find that when you tune in to your body, when you really listen, you can get insights and awareness that lead you toward the pain relief you're seeking.

We live in a culture that is very "head"-centric, very "brain"-centric. We think about everything, analyze everything, try to use logic to get the answers to our most pressing problems, and thus, sadly, we tend to avoid or ignore the body's innate wisdom. When we move out of our heads and into our hearts, our guts, and the body's other centers of knowing, we can find tremendous clarity about our pain, our lives, and how to heal.

We'll begin that process now by looking at a common cause of stress that can be important to address first—feelings of being overwhelmed by your pain, your body, and your life.

Moving into Our Guts—It's Not Just Woo-Woo!

Most of us don't realize how closely connected our guts and brains are. One UCLA study found that gut health has a huge impact on brain function. Study participants (36 women, ages 18–55) were divided into three groups and given fMRI brain scans before and after the study. The first group ate yogurt packed with probiotics, which are central to gut health, twice a day for one month. The second group was given a yogurt-like product that contained no probiotics for the same period of time, and the third group (control group) ate no product at all. At the end of that month, the first group showed changes in several areas of their brains, including emotional as well as sensory processing. So when we talk about "moving into our guts," we're also talking about feeling better emotionally and improving how the body and brain function.

Quieting the Feeling of Being Overwhelmed

I know you're in so much pain that making it through the day with the least possible pain consumes most of your time and energy. How can you possibly do everything you need to do each day when you're in so much pain? You may need more support but hesitate to ask family and friends for help—again. When you're constantly in pain or even wondering when the pain will return, just living your life—managing relationships, finances, doctors, and more—can feel like too much to handle every day.

Feeling overwhelmed can put significant stress on your body. But before we look at the different kinds of stress you may feel, as well as the specific stressors in your life, we first need to quiet, or at least lessen, this overriding sense of feeling overwhelmed. Let's do that now.

First, think about your life. Think about your pain, and everything you need to do every day to manage your pain. Think about your relationships, bills, doctors, medical insurance coverage—all the areas of your life that need your attention. Think about how exhausted you feel and how much more support you need. Really focus on all of it. Let yourself go to that place where you feel totally overwhelmed by this tidal wave of to-dos screaming for your attention. Even reading this book may be adding to your general sense of feeling overwhelmed. What if tapping doesn't work for you? How can you fit tapping into your schedule? It all feels impossible when the pain just won't go away.

When you think about all of these things at once, how overwhelmed do you feel? Give it a number on a scale of 0 to 10. Also make a point of noticing how your pain feels when you're this overwhelmed. Has it shifted in any way? Give your pain its own number, separate from the number you gave your feeling of being overwhelmed.

Next, take a moment to create a picture in your mind. What does feeling overwhelmed look like for you? Create a picture of yourself in your mind with all the mental clutter attached . . . like sticky notes stuck all over your body with reminders of the tasks that need to be done, or your list of "shoulds." How does that picture make you feel? Here, I'll start you out with a list: heavy, full, suffocating, restricted, burdened, helpless, resentful . . . Now it's your turn. Take out your journal and write this all down.

Now let's start tapping:

Karate Chop: Even though I'm feeling overwhelmed with so much to do, I deeply and completely accept myself now.

Karate Chop: Even though I feel the pressure to get it all done, I accept myself and these feelings.

Karate Chop: Even though I have an endless list of things to do, and it's overwhelming, I accept myself now and choose to find a way to feel calm.

Eyebrow: I have so much to do . . .

Side of Eye: It's overwhelming!

Under Eye: And I have to get it all done.

Under Nose: All this pressure to get it all done . . .

Chin: I don't know how I'm going to do it.

Collarbone: It's too much pressure.

Under Arm: It's exhausting.

Top of Head: All these things are screaming for my attention.

Eyebrow: There is so much to do . . .

Side of Eye: I need more support.

Under Eye: It's overwhelming!

Under Nose: I can't relax about this.

Chin: There's so much to do and it's up to me to do it.

Collarbone: It's too much pressure.

Under Arm: I don't know how I'm going to get it all done.

Top of Head: This overwhelming pressure to do it all . . .

Check in with yourself; notice how you're feeling emotionally and how your physical pain is. Keep tapping on the "negative" until the intensity is a 5 or lower, and then switch to some positive rounds. Remember, these "scripts" are just here for guidance and to get you started. Feel free to use your own language, speak your own truth, and so forth.

Positive Round

Eyebrow: I choose to find a way to see this differently.

Side of Eye: Finding a way to let go of this pressure . . .

Under Eye: I take it one step at a time.

Under Nose: Knowing it doesn't have to happen all at once . . .

Chin: Noticing how much lighter it feels . . .

Collarbone: Enjoying the freedom this choice gives me . . .

Under Arm: Letting the pressure melt away . . .

Top of Head: And choosing to feel calm now.

Take a deep breath, and think again about all the things you need to do or tend to. How overwhelmed do you feel now? Give it a number on a scale of 0 to 10. Keep tapping until this feeling is a 3 or lower—even if it takes 20 minutes of tapping. Also take a moment to notice your pain. Did it shift as you were tapping, or after? Give it a number on a scale of 0 to 10. If it changed in any way during this exercise, make note of it. Your body may be trying to tell you that your feeling overwhelmed is linked to your pain in some way.

General Tapping vs. Tapping on Specific Issues

In the last chapter, we learned about the importance of being as specific as possible when you tap. So why are we now tapping on general issues like stress and feeling overwhelmed? While most people do need to dive deeper and get specific about their issues to get lasting pain relief, we often don't know what our specific issues are when we begin tapping. This is where general tapping comes in. Because tapping is so good at initiating the body's relaxation response, by tapping on general issues like stress and feeling overwhelmed, we're better able to get clarity on the more specific areas that need our attention.

Now that we've done some tapping to alleviate your feelings of being overwhelmed, it's time to take a look at stress itself and how different kinds of stress may be affecting you physically and emotionally.

A Fresh Look at Stress

Stress is bad for you. Stress weakens your immune system. Stress may even be contributing to your pain. Every time we look at the news (or pick up a book), there seems to be another negative fact or statistic about stress. It's no wonder that in addition to feeling stress about different issues in our lives—pain, work, relationships, money, and so on—we also feel stressed about being stressed.

But what if our beliefs about stress were more harmful than the stress we feel? In one study, researchers tracked 30,000 adults in the United States over a period of eight years. They began the study by asking participants two questions. First they asked, how much stress have you experienced in the past year? Next they asked, do you believe that stress is harmful to your health? Researchers then tracked public death records to see who died over the next eight years.

They found that the people who had high levels of stress and also believed that stress was harmful to their health had a 43 percent higher risk of premature death—a significantly higher rate than those people who had high levels of stress but believed that stress was a normal part of life. That would mean that just by believing that stress does not harm your health, you could improve your health! That's a completely new way to look at stress.

We spend so much time making stress the enemy that we forget to notice that everyone experiences it. How many people do you know who have zero stress in their lives? I'm guessing none. The best thing you can do is stop worrying about your stress and accept that it's a normal part of life. The bottom line is that we've got to be careful not to pile stress on top of stress. If we're stressing out about being stressed, it just makes matters worse. So, yes, we're looking to reduce the stress in our bodies and our lives, and, yes, stress has significant effects on our physiology and pain, but let's not add to our burden by stressing about it!

Let's do some tapping on that. Say the following sentence out loud and rate how true it feels on a scale of 0 to 10: "I'm stressed out about my stress!" Saying a statement out loud is a great way to "test" how true it feels. Now start tapping:

Karate Chop: Even though it might be true that stress is harmful to my health, I deeply and completely accept myself.

Karate Chop: Even though I've been told that I shouldn't have any stress because it's harmful to my health, I accept myself and my feelings.

Karate Chop: Even though I'm supposed to avoid stress because it's bad for me and sometimes I'm stressing out about stress, I choose to be open-minded to a new idea.

Eyebrow: Stress might be bad for me.

Side of Eye: I'm supposed to avoid stress.

Under Eye: I can't figure out how to avoid stress.

Under Nose: I'm stressed just trying to find a way to avoid it.

Chin: I can't figure out how to avoid stress!

Collarbone: And that's stressful, too.

Under Arm: Feeling stressed is unavoidable . . .

Top of Head: I don't know how to avoid feeling stress.

Check in with yourself and notice how you're feeling emotionally and how your physical pain is. Where is your stress now on a scale of 0 to 10? Keep tapping on the "negative" until the intensity is a 5 or lower, and then switch to some positive rounds. Remember, these "scripts" are just here for guidance and to get you started. Feel free to use your own language, speak your own truth, and so forth.

Positive Round

Eyebrow: I choose to know that stress is manageable.

Side of Eye: I choose to put my attention on things within my control.

Under Eye: I easily find a way to feel more calm.

Under Nose: No matter what is happening around me.

Chin: I calm my reaction by taking a deep breath.

Collarbone: I decide to notice what I am grateful for.

Under Arm: I love knowing that I can change the way I feel.

Top of Head: I can choose to be calm in any situation.

Take a deep breath and check in with yourself again. Now say that sentence aloud: "I'm stressed out about my stress!" On a scale of 0 to 10, how true does that feel now? Keep tapping until you can say that phrase out loud and it rings true at an intensity level of 3 or lower.

Chronic Stress vs. Healthy Stress

Now, all this doesn't mean that stress is good for you, either! The reality is, there are different kinds of stress and we need to be clearer about what we're experiencing exactly. We already looked at one study that suggested that our beliefs about stress are crucial to how stress impacts the body. Other studies suggest that some stress may be good for your health, improving brain function, making you more creative, helping you get fit, and lowering your risk of breast cancer, Alzheimer's, and lots more. What isn't good for your health is chronic stress, the stress that weighs you down and tires you out day after day, month after month, putting you at greater risk for chronic pain.

You've probably experienced these different kinds of stress in your own life. For instance, maybe there have been times when you've had to complete a project that made you nervous but also excited at the same time. The overall experience of getting the project done may have been challenging—and, yes, stressful—but in the end, the time and effort you invested in the project felt really worthwhile. That's an example of healthy stress because it motivated you to accomplish something that was ultimately very rewarding. Once the project was done, your stress levels decreased, and you moved on to a new project.

We also experience healthy stress when we go to the gym and lift heavy weights or run fast, pushing our bodies to grow and adapt. It's uncomfortable in the moment, but we feel great afterward and our bodies reap the rewards.

Chronic stress is different. That's the stress that wears you down. It's as if you spent your whole life in the gym, lifting weights 24/7! That would not be healthy for your body. It's often the "big stuff" in our lives, the puzzles we can't seem to solve—like pain, money, and relationship issues. Science has shown that chronic stress does have a harmful impact on your body. Here's what happens in your body when you're under chronic stress:

1. You think about a topic that often stresses you out, such as your pain, work, money, relationships, family, or something else.

2. Your amygdala (in your midbrain) senses danger.

3. Your amygdala helps to initiate your body's fight-or-flight response to stress.

4. In fight-or-flight mode, your body releases adrenaline and the stress hormone cortisol and diverts blood away from your digestive tract, leaving you less able to digest food and absorb nutrients *and* more likely to gain weight.

5. In this physiological "crisis mode," your muscles are oxygen deprived, which makes you more vulnerable to pain—from chronic illness, injuries, arthritis, fibromyalgia, migraines, stomach upset, and more.

6. In this state of heightened physiological alert, your brain's creative center is deemed nonessential and shuts down. Down go your problem solving, your creative skills, your intuition, your ability to connect with your body.

7. You feel increasingly irritable, isolated, and impatient. Your relationships suffer. Your pain won't go away.

8. Stress affects your sleep. Your metabolism slows. Your body takes longer to heal.

9. Your body secretes even more cortisol, continuing the cycle of oxygen deprivation that contributes to your pain. It also wreaks more havoc on your digestion (and waistline), increases your blood pressure, and lowers your immune response.

10. After releasing too much cortisol for too long, your body goes into adrenal fatigue. You feel depleted, exhausted, and depressed. Your pain is now chronic.

11. You no longer have the energy to adhere to your exercise routine, your healthy eating, meditation, or yoga. Chronic pain seems to be running your life.

12. Your energy is low, and you have a hard time focusing. Your productivity declines further. Your relationships suffer. You're still in pain.

13. You are *stressed out*. You feel depressed. Your muscles are chronically tense and oxygen deprived, making your chronic pain even more intense and more frequent. You need relief—from your pain and your stress—now.

That paints a pretty gloomy picture of what chronic stress does to you and your body. So what's the final verdict—is stress normal or harmful?

The Final Verdict on Stress

Is stress a normal part of life that only hurts you if you believe it's harmful? Or is chronic stress escalating your pain and harming your health?

While there are many different ways to look at stress, both of the viewpoints we've looked at so far are valid. We all have stress in our lives. Worrying about that stress only increases it, and that doesn't serve anyone. The fact that you're in chronic pain, however, suggests that chronic stress isn't serving you, either. And since tapping is an incredibly powerful tool for stress relief (and pain relief), it's a powerful asset for decreasing the "bad" (chronic) stress in your life so you can get in touch with your body and accelerate the pain-relief process.

We'll continue that process now by looking at the frustration so many people feel when they're in pain.

Romantic Love and Pain Relief

In one study conducted at Stanford University, 15 study participants were examined via fMRI during the first nine months of new romantic relationships. All the study participants completed three tasks while being subjected to moderate to intense thermal pain: (1) looked at a photo of their romantic partner; (2) looked at a picture of an equally attractive and familiar acquaintance; (3) did a word-association distraction task that had previously been shown to reduce pain. Both the first task (viewing a photo of their romantic partner) and the third (word-association task demonstrated to provide pain relief) reduced pain, but only when they were looking at a photo of their partner did several reward-processing areas of the brain become activated. Those findings suggest that intense feelings of romantic love may provide or increase pain relief in the body.

Facing the Frustration

When I'm working with groups of pain clients, whether at an event or on the phone, people often get frustrated when one person gets an incredible result and they don't. They've tried so many different pain-relief remedies, but none has worked. Why would tapping be any different?

Instead of trying to push that frustration aside, we need to stop and acknowledge the stress and strain it's putting on our bodies. We need to accept that frustration for what it is and acknowledge that it's keeping us stuck. The white pill mentality has made us think that X is the cure for Y. But with chronic pain, it's not so simple. And laying out that understanding for ourselves is healthy and important. Everyone is different. We each need to acknowledge ourselves as unique and be willing to have different experiences with pain relief. The fact that one person got pain relief in their first hour of tapping doesn't mean the tapping you've been doing for two weeks isn't working. It means that your pain-relief journey is unique to you.

I know that accepting your pain-relief journey, which may not yet have provided the pain relief you're seeking, is a lot easier said than done. You want to get rid of the pain now. You want to fix your body (and your life) now. The frustration you feel because that hasn't happened yet is normal. But that frustration is also something you need to really face and begin to release through tapping. I know you want to focus on the pain, not on your frustration, but you can't afford to ignore or deny the frustration anymore, because that frustration is building. As it builds, it's creating more stress in your body. And as we've seen, by not expressing that emotion—your frustration—you may be interfering with your own pain relief.

So let's do some tapping now on all the frustration you feel about your pain, about the different pain-relief options you've tried that haven't worked, about having to try yet another form of pain relief. Facing your frustration may feel overwhelming at first, as if it's more than you can handle when you're in all this pain, but your feeling that you'll crumble under the weight of your frustration is an indication of how much you need to express it.

Take a moment now to really tune in to your frustration. Really let yourself feel it. On a scale of 0 to 10, how frustrated do you feel? How much pain do you feel? Give it a separate number on a scale of 0 to 10. Write these both in your journal. Now let's start tapping:

Karate Chop: Even though I am so frustrated with this pain, I deeply and completely accept myself.

Karate Chop: Even though I've tried so many things to get rid of the pain and I am still dealing with it, and it's so frustrating, I choose to accept myself now.

Karate Chop: Even though I have all this pain frustration in my life, I accept my feelings and choose to release the frustration.

Eyebrow: This pain is so frustrating.

Side of Eye: I've tried so many things to heal it . . .

Under Eye: And nothing has worked.

Under Nose: It's so frustrating . . .

Chin: Now this is one more thing.

Collarbone: And what if it doesn't work . . .

Under Arm: I'm so tired of this pain!

Top of Head: It's one frustrating thing after another.

Eyebrow: It takes up so much of my time.

Side of Eye: It takes up so much of my life.

Under Eye: I want my life back.

Under Nose: It's so frustrating!

Chin: Nothing I do seems to help . . .

Collarbone: I don't want to be disappointed again.

Under Arm: I'm afraid to try one more thing . . .

Top of Head: This frustration never seems to go away.

Check in with yourself and notice how you feel emotionally and how your pain is. Keep tapping on the "negative" until the intensity is a 5 or lower and then switch to some positive rounds. Remember, these scripts are just here for guidance and to get you started. Feel free to use your own language, speak your own truth, and so forth.

Positive Round

Eyebrow: I'm ready to give this tapping a chance . . .

Side of Eye: What if this makes a big difference . . .

Under Eye: I choose a higher quality of life . . .

Under Nose: I choose to clear this pain in my body . . .

Chin: I choose to do my best now.

Collarbone: I do this for me.

Under Arm: I choose to accept progress . . .

Top of Head: I choose to know that I'm making a difference.

Take a deep breath and check in with yourself. On a scale of 0 to 10, how frustrated do you feel now? Keep tapping until your frustration is a 3 or lower. Notice also if your pain shifted during or after tapping on your frustration. If so, make a note of it. That may mean that your pain is connected to your frustration in some way.

Releasing Old Patterns That Create Chronic Stress

"I'm not sure I'm doing it right." "My mind wanders while I'm tapping." "I know I need to tap every day, but I never seem to get to it." We're all so worried about doing everything perfectly that we sabotage our attempts to move forward. Every time a client says something like this to me, I remind them that the patterns that helped to get them to where they are now won't help them get rid of their pain. So, for example, if you've always put a lot of pressure on yourself to do everything perfectly, that pattern of perfectionism won't help you get the pain relief you're seeking. You're going to have to establish new, healthier patterns!

• •

The patterns that have helped you get to where you are now won't help you get rid of your pain. If you've always put a lot of pressure on yourself to do everything perfectly, that pattern of perfectionism won't help you get the pain relief you're seeking . . . It's time to establish new, healthier patterns of behavior and thinking!

• •

One of the great things about tapping is that you don't have to do it perfectly for it to work. By putting pressure on yourself to tap "better" or more often, you're creating more stress that may then interfere with your pain relief. To move forward in this pain-relief process, you need to begin noticing patterns like perfectionism that may be creating chronic stress in your life. Then you can use tapping to overcome them and move forward in a new way.

While perfectionism is one of the most common patterns I see in clients, there are many different patterns that can create chronic stress. During a Q & A call I hosted a few weeks after a pain-relief event, Becky shared that she was having a hard time motivating herself to tap, even though tapping had lowered her pain at the event. When she explained in more detail what was going on in her life, it was clear that Becky was stuck in an old pattern of keeping herself busy at all times.

She knew she needed to slow down and take better care of herself, but she found herself constantly making more commitments than she could handle, especially given her chronic pain. In the days before our call, Becky had kept herself so busy that she'd fallen down three separate times and gotten a black eye. Since falling, her pain had increased. She said that by pressuring herself to do so much, she felt as if she was literally "beating herself up," but she didn't know how to stop.

We did some tapping on learning how to put less pressure on herself, and after a few minutes, she said she felt more relaxed and willing to do less in order to feel better. She could see how her pattern of always needing to be extremely busy was working against her. While I was happy that she had gotten that clarity, knowing how ingrained patterns like these often are, I decided to challenge her further.

"So what if it takes a year of using tapping for maybe an hour a week to get rid of your pain?" I asked.

"That's way too long! I can't wait another whole year!" she replied, clearly agitated by the thought of having to wait that long.

"Okay, so what if I tell you that you can either keep running around, staying as busy as ever, and still be in pain a year from now, or you can stop putting so much pressure on yourself, focus on relieving your pain with tapping at a slower pace, and be able to look back a year from now and not have any pain? Which one would you choose?"

Silence.

"I guess the last one—for it to take a year to get rid of my pain," she answered. "But it still feels like too long."

By the end of the call, she'd agreed to put less pressure on herself and to make a plan to add tapping into her schedule consistently but in a way that was manageable.

Let me say this again because it's really important. Patterns like perfectionism and overdoing are hard to break. It takes time and attention to create new and healthier patterns. Even after you've gotten out of them, you may occasionally fall into old patterns and then catch yourself and have to course correct over time. That's okay. What's important is that you begin to pay attention to the patterns in your life that aren't serving you, the patterns that are creating chronic stress.

Identify Your Stress Pattern

In your journal, write down three things that cause you to stress. (I know there may be more, but let's start with three for now!)

Now, make a short list of the things you do to avoid feeling the stress, for example, watching TV for hours, raiding the refrigerator, or playing video games for hours.

Now it's time to be honest with yourself. What feelings would come up if you didn't do those things? What feelings do you not want to experience?

I bet you're seeing a pattern already! Tapping can become a positive and powerful tool to release the feelings you have been trying to avoid.

Next, we'll do some tapping on beginning to break this pattern. First, though, check in on your pain, give it a number on a scale of 0 to 10, and write it down in your journal.

Karate Chop: Even though I need this pattern when I get stressed, I deeply and completely accept myself now.

Karate Chop: Even though this pattern helps me when I feel stressed and can't handle it, I can find something new that works just as well.

Karate Chop: Even though I get overwhelmed and stressed and need to escape, and that's why I can't let go of this familiar pattern, I choose to know I am safe now.

Eyebrow: A part of me needs this pattern . . .

Side of Eye: I need it for when I feel stressed . . .

Under Eye: For when I can't handle it anymore . . .

Under Nose: For when I need to escape . . .

Chin: This pattern has kept me safe.

Collarbone: I think I need this pattern.

Under Arm: I'm not sure how to change this pattern.

Top of Head: I want to change this pattern, but I don't know how.

Eyebrow: I'm choosing to feel resourceful.

Side of Eye: What if there were ways to feel calm and comfortable . . .

Under Eye: I've decided to take the pressure off myself . . .

Under Nose: I think it is possible to change this pattern.

Chin: What if it is easier than I thought to change this pattern . . .

Collarbone: I love knowing I don't have to do it right . . .

Under Arm: I only have to do it.

Top of Head: I'm open to enjoying new ways to feel calm.

When you're done, check in with yourself and give your pain a number. Make note of that in your journal, along with any shifts you experienced with your emotions as well as physically.

Managing Everyday Stress

Mark's voice was flat and tight. After he'd gotten rid of his chronic back pain during the tapping event, several weeks had passed, and his pain had begun to come back. It wasn't as severe as it had been before the event, and it only flared up occasionally, but this particular day, he was having a bad day. The middle of his back felt oddly numb; he had a sharp, stabbing pain in his lower back and a burning pain in his upper back. When I asked how he felt about his pain coming back, he said that he felt irritated, especially because the pain had started after he'd bent down to pick up a shirt, a very simple movement that he didn't feel should cause pain. We began by tapping directly on his pain. After several minutes, the stabbing pain in his lower back went down significantly from an 8 to a 2, the numbness went away completely, and his low back pain went from a 5 down to a 1—a huge shift in just minutes.

While I was excited by his results, I sensed that there was more to work through, and I asked him again how he felt and what was going on in his life. He shared that he'd woken up at 3 A.M., as he does every night, shocked awake by what felt like a bolt of electricity running through his body. When I asked him what he thought the electricity was all about, he said he felt anxious.

He then added that he felt stuck in several areas of his life. "Give me one example of an area where you feel stuck," I said.

"Financial matters," he immediately replied. "There are several fairly important things I need to tend to, but when I think about them, I get this feeling of dread. There's just a lot of anxiety around it all."

As we continued talking about money, Mark's back pain went back up to about a 5.

While I never want clients to be in more pain, I actually get excited when there's a shift like that during a session. You can clearly see the link between Mark's back pain and his anxiety around finances. That's really useful information that we can then use to discover the deeper cause of his pain. When I asked Mark if there was anything specifically about money that made him anxious, he said it was financial planning.

We then spent several minutes tapping on his anxiety around finances, specifically around how overwhelmed he felt about planning for the future. As we tapped through the points, we asked questions like "What is this stress around finances all about?" and "What is this pain all about?" In addition to being a powerful tool for resolving issues, tapping is great for uncovering memories and emotions that are still impacting us but that have gotten buried over time. When you come to a question that you can't answer, try asking yourself the question repeatedly while tapping through the points.

After a few minutes of asking himself these questions while tapping, Mark began remembering how his dad had used money to control him and his brother when they were growing up. One memory in particular had come to Mark's mind as he was tapping, bringing with it a lot of fear and anxiety around money.

It was one morning when Mark was 18, soon after he'd returned from an extended trip to Europe. Without saying a word, his dad walked into his room, threw a stack of bills on his bed, and then walked out. Mark didn't know what to make of his dad's gesture. His takeaway was fear. He remembered being terrified of the consequences, unsure if his dad would make him find a way to pay the bills or cut him off financially, or if there would be physical consequences.

I then asked Mark to retell the story while tapping through the points, running through it several times until the intensity of the memory was lower. When he was done, I asked him to imagine meeting with a financial adviser, while continuing to tap through the points. Tapping while bringing up challenging memories or situations in our minds can be really powerful because it helps us to connect with the emotions those memories or situations create in us. Because tapping is so good at relieving stress, people can often process difficult emotions and events without getting overwhelmed.

"What happens if the financial adviser tells you that you've mismanaged your money and you and your family are screwed?" I asked Mark.

"Now I'm not talking to a financial adviser. I'm talking to my dad," he replied insightfully.

Tapping Tip

When you're trying to clear a memory or event, use the Movie Technique (see page 31). While tapping through the points, run the movie of that event, including sights, sounds, smells, and any other details you remember, through your mind over and over again until you can recall it without feeling the emotional charge it once had. That's when you know you've cleared it.

As we continued tapping while doing these visioning exercises, Mark's fear and anxiety turned into anger at his dad for not teaching him what he'd done wrong and what he needed to do better. We continued tapping on his anger, using reminder phrases like "all this anger at my dad" and "all this stress and anger in my back." We did multiple rounds, and then we completed the final rounds with phrases like "I choose to release all this stress and anger in my back now" and "I choose to release all this anger at my dad right now."

When we were done tapping, Mark's back pain and anxiety were gone. I asked him to think about his finances again. "I don't feel any anxiety," he shared. His voice was noticeably more upbeat than it had been at the beginning of our call.

"I actually feel like I want to go get some work done," he then added. Now that he'd relieved some of his anxiety, fear, and anger, Mark was ready to get unstuck in his life and begin dealing with the things he'd been avoiding. That shift, in a matter of minutes, was profound not only for his pain but also for his life.

Sessions like this are powerful reminders of how deeply rooted everyday stressors such as money, relationships, and work often are. When stress and emotions like anxiety and fear become so chronic that they turn into physical pain, we need to stop and look beneath the surface. By exploring the deeper layers of everyday stress through tapping, we often begin to pinpoint bigger areas—the different layers of Mark's relationship with his father, for example—that need more attention. That's the process we'll be doing throughout this book. Let's begin by looking at the things that are stressing you out in your life.

Imagine yourself at the start of your day taking a look forward at all the events and tasks that you've got lined up to do.

See yourself at the first task and put a number from 0 to 10 (where 10 is the most stress) on how stressful you imagine that event to be. Example: getting the kids off to school—7. Write that down in your journal, along with a number rating the intensity of your physical pain when you think about that first stressful task of the day.

What about that event do you anticipate being stressful? Example: "I'm already in pain and the kids aren't cooperating and I'm starting to feel frustrated and impatient."

Do a few minutes of tapping, not worrying about the specific language, just voicing how you feel. It might look like this:

Eyebrow: This is going to be so hard . . .

Side of Eye: It's so much work getting everyone and everything ready in the morning . . .

Under Eye: And I hurt . . .

Under Nose: I'm exhausted . . .

Chin: It's just too much.

Collarbone: I didn't sleep well.

Under Arm: Is it ever going to get easier . . .

Top of Head: Why can't they just listen to me . . .

Eyebrow: I need help with all of this . . .

Side of Eye: It's just too much for my body . . .

Under Eye: I have too much pain.

Under Nose: I can hardly keep it together . . .

Chin: And this is just the start of my day.

Collarbone: I anticipate being in a lot more pain by evening . . .

Under Arm: What if I could release some of this tension . . .

Top of Head: I know this tension is tied to the pain.

Check in with yourself and notice how you're feeling emotionally and how your physical pain is. Give each a number on a scale of 0 to 10. Keep tapping on the "negative" until the intensity is a 5 or lower and then switch to some positive rounds. Remember, these scripts are just here for guidance and to get you started. Feel free to use your own language, speak your own truth, and so forth.

Positive Round

Eyebrow: I can tap for the tension . . .

Side of Eye: I'm choosing to do something good for me.

Under Eye: When I let the tension and stress go . . .

Under Nose: My body feels better . . .

Chin: And when my body feels better . . .

Collarbone: I am a better version of me . . .

Under Arm: And my day goes better.

Top of Head: I choose calm as I start my day.

Take a deep breath and look at it again. On a scale of 0 to 10, what number would you give it now? Continue through the events of the day until you can stand back and look at your day from a much calmer place, ideally until the negative emotional charge is a 3 or lower. Also make a note of any shifts you experience in your pain.

Creating a New Relationship with Your Body

As we've seen, there's often no clear line between physical pain and emotional and psychic pain. The pain-relief process laid out in this book doesn't just treat physical pain; it treats everything that comes with it. The frustration, angst, anger, sadness; the thoughts of a life lost, of what could be, of relationships damaged; and the loss of physical function, good health, autonomy, and more are all critical aspects of this process. We will explore all of those layers, but first we need to release stress and get reconnected to the body.

In many ways you may feel like your body has betrayed you, imprisoning you in pain and preventing you from living the life you know is still possible. Like I said before, I understand that getting connected with your body may be the last thing you want to do, because this is where you feel the pain most. But it's time to make peace with your body. It's time to begin listening to what your body and your pain are trying to tell you. Let's do some tapping now on reconnecting with your body.

Take a moment to think about listening to your body. How much resistance do you feel? Give it a number on a scale of 0 to 10. Also make a point of noticing how your pain feels when you think about reconnecting with your body. Give your pain its own number, separate from the number you gave your resistance. Note these in your journal and then start tapping:

Karate Chop: Even though I don't want to get connected with this painful body, I still choose to accept myself.

Karate Chop: Even though my body is not my friend right now, I can still choose to accept myself and my body.

Karate Chop: Even though this body hasn't worked right and I have all these feelings about it, I can accept that this is how I feel about my body right now.

Eyebrow: I don't want to connect with this body . . .

Side of Eye: This body is letting me down.

Under Eye: This body and all its limitations . . .

Under Nose: It's keeping me from doing so many things . . .

Chin: This body holds me prisoner . . .

Collarbone: It would take a lot of work to connect with this body.

Under Arm: I don't know how to connect with my body.

Top of Head: It's not safe to connect with my body.

Check in with yourself and rate the intensity on a scale of 0 to 10. Keep tapping on the "negative" until the intensity is a 5 or lower and then switch to some positive rounds. Remember, these scripts are just here for guidance and to get you started. Feel free to use your own language, speak your own truth, and so forth.

Positive Rounds

Eyebrow: Maybe I can begin to think about connecting with my body . . .

Side of Eye: Maybe my body has been doing its best to protect me.

Under Eye: This body has gone through a lot . . .

Under Nose: And it's doing its best to heal.

Chin: My body wants to feel good . . .

Collarbone: I want my body to feel good.

Under Arm: What if I started to accept my body right now . . .

Top of Head: What if my body and I started to work together . . .

Eyebrow: Perhaps I can connect with my body . . .

Side of Eye: What if we were healing together . . .

Under Eye: I want to give my body another chance . . .

Under Nose: I know my body wants to feel good . . .

Chin: I want to feel good.

Collarbone: I choose to connect with my body now . . .

Under Arm: To be accepting of myself and my body . . .

Top of Head: We are on this journey to healing together.

Take a deep breath and think again about listening to your body. How much resistance do you feel now? Give it a number on a scale of 0 to 10. Keep tapping until your resistance, and any other negative emotional charge, is a 3 or lower—even if it takes 20 minutes of tapping. Also notice any shifts you experience in your pain.

Amazing Results Can Happen to Anyone!

Vickie had attended all three days of my live pain-relief event, and she had bravely come up onstage to tell her story and share her challenges. While she'd left the event with the pain still in her back, instead of coming away with nothing, as she'd expected, she went home with something she felt was really important, something that could easily be overlooked because of its simplicity but that had profound effects for her.

For the first time since her diagnosis, which had been delivered rudely and with a cruel footnote that her condition would eventually land her in a wheelchair, she shared, "I went home [from the event] with a sliver of hope." During a Q & A call a few weeks later, she updated me on her progress. "If all those people got those kinds of results [from tapping], then surely there's hope for me. Giving up is not even in my vocabulary anymore."

Taking a cue from hearing how determined she sounded, I asked her how her back pain was in that moment. She said it was an 8 out of 10. "Okay, tell me what's going on for you. What's happening in your life?" I asked. She said that she had been feeling overwhelmed and was having difficulty focusing when she tapped. She also shared that in spite of her hope, she felt frustrated that she hadn't yet experienced pain relief from tapping. When I asked her if she'd be willing to do some tapping on that frustration itself, she quickly replied, "Sure!"

We did several rounds of tapping on her frustration at still being in pain, even though she had her "sliver of hope." We also tapped on the back pain itself. "That was amazing!" she said after we'd finished. While tapping, she'd felt heat across her back, which she'd never felt before. Minutes later, her pain went away, which she'd never experienced before, either.

"So *this* is what it's like . . . to be one of *those* people who get results . . . It's incredible! I feel incredible. It's like I'm just back from a wonderful weekend away, and I'm back now, and I feel incredible."

I asked if anything had come up for her during the tapping. "No," she replied. "I just really focused in on the frustration. It was just you and me, focusing on my issue. I bring so much heaviness to it all, but you just focused right in on my issue, and now I feel amazing."

What I love about Vickie's story is her determination to stick with the process. Throughout the three-day pain-relief event she attended, she watched other people get great pain-relief results. After each breakthrough, people would stand up, bend over, and twist in the aisle. After tapping, they could easily and painlessly make all the movements they never could make when they were in pain. Vickie had not been one of those people, but she'd held on to her sliver of hope. She kept tapping, and when she least expected it, during a simple Q & A call, she got the results she'd been seeking.

Vickie is such a great example of how different this process is for everyone and how patience and determination can really pay off. The first step in Vickie's pain-relief process was reconnecting with her hope. In doing that, she gave herself and her body the chance to begin to heal and to get back in control of her life.

Also important to note about Vickie's shift, and something you might want to explore yourself, is how the frustration about the problem itself can be what's keeping you stuck. Time and again I've seen how the ongoing frustration can build up on itself and keep someone in pain. Releasing that frustration can be monumental in experiencing a shift.

Your Future Self

This "Future Self" exercise, which you'll see at the end of several chapters, is a simple, thought-provoking way to help you envision a healthier, brighter future.

You can write your answers to these questions in your journal, or just daydream about them.

We'll dive into a process of envisioning and creating your future in more detail later in the book, but as we move forward, this brief exercise will get you thinking about the positive changes you intend to make as a result of this process, not just for pain relief, but throughout your life.

As you answer these questions, tap through the points as you feel, visualize, and imagine these aspects of your "Future Self":

- What will the look on my face be when I'm feeling calm and relaxed?

- What will I notice when I'm feeling less stress?

- Who will notice these changes the most?

Audio Bonus: Download a free audio version of "Tapping on Feeling overwhelmed": thetappingsolution.com/painbookresources.

CHAPTER 4

ADDRESSING THE EMOTIONAL AND PHYSICAL IMPACT OF EVENTS

"What was happening in your life when the pain first started?"

It's an incredibly simple question that few of my clients have ever been asked by a doctor, and sometimes not by a friend or family member, either. They've been poked and prodded, X-rayed, scanned, tested, isolated, and sometimes cut open, but no one ever looked into their eyes and acknowledged that they're more than a collection of cells, muscles, nerves, and bones.

Like you, each of them is a unique person, a complex network of physical cells, nerves, limbs, as well as thoughts, emotions, needs, desires, and experiences that interplay in ways that Western medicine has yet to understand completely. And like you, they have a story that's uniquely their own.

Starting in this chapter and throughout most of the remainder of the book, we'll be focusing on your story. We'll look at your story from different angles and get specific about the different pieces of it so we can process and release the deeper layers of your pain.

To begin that process, we'll start by focusing on what was happening in your life when the pain began and on the emotional impact of these events. It's one of the first questions I ask clients because it's a powerful way to begin retracing the steps of your journey.

Different Kinds of "Events"

To fully understand how events can impact pain, we first need to define *event.* The way I talk about events is often much wider than just a onetime occurrence. From my experiences, I've figured out that there are two distinct kinds of events that can initiate pain. For some people, the pain began with a *physical event,* like an accident or injury. Other people begin experiencing pain for reasons that aren't as obvious, such as an emotionally charged time in their life or a specific emotional trauma. I refer to these as *emotional events.*

So let's begin to explore what was happening in your life when your pain began, looking at the full spectrum of events in your life at that time. Even if your pain began with a physical event, like an injury or accident, it's important that you do this exercise and look back at that time in your life from multiple angles. As we'll see, it's often the mix of emotional and physical events and circumstances that creates chronic pain.

Take a moment now to get your journal and, if possible, find a quiet place where you can really focus. Close your eyes, if that feels comfortable, and tap through the points as you remember what was happening in your life when the pain began. Then, when you're ready, open your eyes and write down everything that came to mind. It can be helpful to tap while remembering what happened because it calms the body and often helps our subconscious mind bring new ideas, memories, thoughts, and feelings to the surface.

Next, look through the list of questions below and write your answers down in your journal. If any of your answers are already included in the journal entry you just made, skip to the next question. If you're finding it difficult to remember, try tapping through the points while asking yourself each question repeatedly and see what comes up.

- What was happening in your work/financial life?
- What was happening in your relationship?
- What was happening in your family?

- What was happening in your home?

- What was happening with friends?

- What was happening with your health?

- What was happening in your body?

- What else was happening in your life at that time?

When you're done writing down everything you remember from that time, read through what you've written. Leave extra white space in that part of your journal for anything you may remember later. A bit later in the chapter, we'll do some tapping on what you've written down. First, however, we'll take a look at how your emotional state may affect your body's ability to heal from physical events and then explore how events can contribute to chronic pain.

The Power of Physical Events

When I first asked Nicole to raise her right arm, she hesitated but then tried it. Once her arm was a few inches away from the side of her body, she winced and lowered it. "It's frozen," she explained, referring to her right shoulder. It had been very painful for almost three years, since she'd injured it while doing repetitive overhead work. Remembering that time, she added, "I was basically working myself into my own grave." Since the injury, her life had been severely limited by her shoulder pain. "Some days, all I can do is lie down," she shared in a sad, quiet voice. Since the injury, she'd also undergone two shoulder surgeries, but she still hadn't gotten the pain relief and mobility she desperately wanted.

Nicole had volunteered to come up onstage and share her story during an event in Melbourne, Australia. When I asked how intense her shoulder pain was, she said it was a 7 out of 10. She also had neurological pain that radiated down from her neck, she added.

We began with some general tapping, focusing on "all this pain in my body." While doing a few rounds of tapping, Nicole felt a sudden jolt of pain, and immediately afterward, her pain moved down to under her arm. The intensity was slightly lower, she said, now a 6 out of 10. I asked her to try raising her arm again, and she got it about an inch higher than she had only a few minutes before.

Now that Nicole was feeling slightly more relaxed, I asked her what emotion she felt was in her shoulder. "Worry, I guess?" she replied. "What's the worry about?" I asked. "About my pain, and the fact that I've been in pain for so long and can't see the light at the end of the tunnel. I just want it gone so I can get on with my life," she said.

We then began tapping, focusing on "all this worry in my shoulder," "this frozen shoulder," and "all this fear and anxiety that my pain won't go away." After several rounds, I asked what had shifted. She smiled. "I'm just tingling," she said. She then lifted her arms two or three inches higher than she had the last time. "It's still very painful," she said, "but there's definitely energy moving in my arm. I can feel it." Her pain had gone down another notch, to a 5 out of 10. Her shoulder was still hurting, but I could see the excitement on her face.

Next I asked her to tap through the points while telling the story of what happened at the time of her injury, focusing on emotions, as well as sights, smells, sounds, and colors, from that time. This is the Movie Technique we learned in Chapter 2, and it's a great way to bring up and process memories and emotions from the past. The basic idea here is to tap as you're talking, which allows you to connect to the stuck energy, trauma, and emotions from that time. By allowing yourself to feel and voice it while tapping, you're able to release it.

Before telling even a word of her story, she began crying quietly. As she tapped, she shared that, before her injury, she'd been working in her dream job as a purser on a cruise ship. Her mom had become ill, however, and she'd had to quit that job and work instead at an agency, doing odd jobs and working long hours to make up the money she'd lost on the cruise ship. Her mom then developed dementia, and Nicole had been forced to take care of her while also working intense hours. "It was a very emotional and stressful time," she explained. "I had no help, and I was caring for my mom while also suffering and in pain and also working a lot of hours . . . It feels better just talking about it," she added.

We began tapping on the trauma she'd experienced during that time and how it had stayed with her in her frozen shoulder. After just one round of tapping, she shared that her entire right side had become hot. "It's hot pain," she said, "but something's moving." She then raised her arm even higher, another couple of inches higher than the time before. She smiled and laughed, almost giddy with amazement.

With her pain still a 5 out of 10, I knew it was time to go deeper. "What's really going on with this pain and your frozen shoulder?" I asked. "What's the emotional significance of this pain and this frozen shoulder?" She swallowed hard and shared that she'd had a lot of hurt from her mother and from her family.

"When I was caring for Mom, I really had no help from anybody," she explained. I asked her how she felt now about her family and the fact that they hadn't helped her at all during her mother's illness. "I've forgiven everyone," she immediately said. "Has your shoulder forgiven them?" I asked. She laughed. "I don't know," she replied.

We then did several rounds of tapping, beginning with the setup statement "Even though I've forgiven everybody, though maybe my shoulder hasn't, I deeply and completely love and accept myself." We tapped on her anger and rage at her family for not helping her, for how they treated her. We also tapped on releasing that anger and rage, on unfreezing her shoulder, and on letting go of the pain.

As we were finishing the final tapping round, she began opening and closing her hand. "What was happening there?" I asked her once we'd finished. "It went cold. It's not hot anymore. It's cold and tingly. Something's happening here," she replied, laughing as relief visibly washed over her face.

In just 20 minutes, her shoulder pain had gone down significantly, she'd been able to raise her hand to a 45-degree angle for the first time since her injury, and she'd pinpointed the true source of her pain—her anger and rage at her family for not helping her during her mother's illness and dementia. I asked her if she'd thought she could keep tapping on that time, on releasing her anger and rage. She happily nodded yes. If just that small amount of tapping had cut her shoulder pain almost in half, there's a good chance she can get rid of it altogether if she keeps tapping.

Watch Nicole's Session, Live! You can watch a video of this session and tap along here: thetappingsolution.com/painbookresources.

Let's quickly take a look at the process I guided Nicole through to drill down to the core emotions behind her "frozen shoulder":

1. I had her tell me what was going on in her body, the story behind her pain.

2. We checked in on her pain and she gave it a number from 0 to 10.

3. We tapped directly on the pain sensations she was feeling.

4. We checked in on her pain to see if it had shifted, which it had, going from a 7 out of 10 down to a 6 out of 10.

5. I began to dig deeper into the emotions behind the pain by asking her what emotion was in her "frozen shoulder."

6. We then tapped on the emotion, which in her case was worry.

7. We checked in on her pain again, which had now gone down to a 5 out of 10.

8. I had her tell the story of her pain while tapping through the points. Because clients have done some initial tapping by this point, they're more relaxed, so this is often when we can go deep and discover the true source of their pain.

9. We checked in on the pain again, which was still a 5 out of 10. Since there had been no movement, I asked her to continue tapping as I asked a probing question—what's really going on with this pain?

10. As she began sharing the deeper layers of her story—the fact that her other family members hadn't offered her any help caring for her mom—we identified anger as the true source of her pain and tapped until her pain was almost entirely gone.

When we're processing emotional events like these, we need to remember that tapping isn't an eraser tool. We don't just tap for a few rounds and suddenly the frozen shoulder is gone forever. What's so powerful about tapping is that it allows you to feel the emotion(s), feel the pain, and, through the tapping process, connect to the emotions and energy that have gotten stuck in the body. That process can take time.

I was reminded of the importance of this process one day while interviewing Louise Hay for my company's annual Tapping World Summit. As we were discussing tapping, and how it requires that we look at the "negative"—challenges we're facing within ourselves and in our lives—I asked her, "You believe more than anyone in the world about being positive, but why is it important to take a look at what's happening?" In her typically warm and comforting way, she replied, "If you're going to clean a house, you have to see the dirt. If you're going to clean a turkey pan, if you're going to do the dishes, you have to see the dirt that you're cleaning. When you do that, then you can do lots of good affirmations." And she's right. When we tap on what happened when the pain first began, we're beginning to clean the house on several levels—emotionally and energetically as well as physically. That "cleaning house" process is essentially what we'll be doing throughout this book. While I realize that letting yourself feel challenging emotions, as well as your pain, isn't always appealing, as we've seen, allowing yourself to "go there" is a critical part of the pain-relief process.

What's so powerful about tapping is that it allows you to feel the emotion(s), feel the pain, and, through the tapping process, connect to the emotions and energy that have gotten stuck in the body. That process can take time.

The Equation for Pain

When we're discussing physical events like Nicole's, looking at how emotions contributed to pain, it can be easy to assume that emotions are the true cause of chronic pain. That's not necessarily the case. In most cases, it's not a single factor that is responsible for chronic pain. So, for instance, it's not that you were having stress in your life, so your back started to hurt. It's the combination of circumstances that often leads to pain. So your pain may have started and then become chronic because your stress levels were high, which wears down your body. Then you made a movement and pulled your back. It hurt, and so you got scared about your back, which made your body more vulnerable—and the cycle continues.

All these different factors—your movements, your emotions, what was happening in your life, and much more—are what add up to chronic pain. They become an equation for chronic pain. So, for example, while someone doing the same repetitive work Nicole was doing might have also injured their shoulder, without the stress and emotional turmoil Nicole was feeling, that other person's shoulder might have fully healed within a few weeks, leaving them with no pain and full mobility.

This concept of an equation for chronic pain is important because it helps to take some of the blame off ourselves. While your emotions may have contributed to your pain, it's important for you to understand that your pain is not your fault. You didn't "ask for it," and there's nothing inherently wrong with you, your emotions, your life, or your body. Negative emotions are a normal and natural part of the human experience, and the cause of your chronic pain is not just negative thinking or genetics or poor decisions or any one thing. It's more like a perfect storm, a specific combination of physical, mental, and emotional circumstances that came together and created chronic pain.

Fortunately, by going through this process of peeling back the different layers that created the pain, we can find the perfect combination of techniques for undoing the effects of that original "perfect storm." So, for example, your perfect combination for overcoming chronic pain for good might be tapping to release emotions and energy that have gotten stuck in your body, as well as better nutrition, regular exercise, the right medical help, and so on. Each of us is unique, so your goal is to keep using tapping to explore your story from different angles so you can figure out your perfect combination for putting an end to chronic pain.

Tapping on a Physical Event

If your pain began with a physical event, like an injury or accident, take a moment now to do this tapping exercise. If your pain did not begin with a physical event, you can skip to the next section of this chapter, "Unpeeling the Layers of Emotional Events."

Take a moment now to close your eyes and think back to what happened. How intense is the emotional charge of that memory? Give it a number on a scale of 0 to 10. Write this down in your journal.

While tapping through the points, tell the story, including all the details you remember. Try to include everything that was happening during that time, so if your work, relationship, or family was a big source of stress around the time your physical event took place, make sure to tap on those emotional components in addition to the physical event itself.

Note: If the event was especially traumatic, and you don't feel comfortable tapping through it on your own, I encourage you to seek out the support of an EFT practitioner first. You can find a list at thetappingsolution.com/eft-practitioners.

Here's an example of what this tapping might look like as you "tell the story":

Eyebrow: We were on our way to the movies . . .
Side of Eye: I was driving and my sister was sitting in the front seat.

Under Eye: It was raining pretty hard.

Under Nose: I had just changed lanes to get in the lane for the next exit . . .

Chin: And this little Toyota came zooming up beside me . . .

Collarbone: And there was no place for me to go.

(*Note:* As an example, you might find that you feel more of a charge here when you say, "There was no place for me to go." You can keep tapping on that phrase until the intensity goes down. If, at any point, it doesn't feel safe to tap, reach out to a trained practitioner.)

Under Arm: There was no place for me to go.

Top of Head: There was no place for me to go.

Eyebrow: There was no place for me to go.

Side of Eye: There was nothing I could do.

Under Eye: I knew we were going to hit . . .

Under Nose: And there was no place for me to go.

Chin: There was nothing I could do . . .

Collarbone: I was so scared.

Under Arm: There was no place for me to go.

Top of Head: I knew we were going to hit, and there was no place for me to go.

Now, without tapping, go back and watch the movie up to that point, saying those words again. When you get to the part where you say, "There was no place for me to go," notice how it feels. Give it a number on a scale of 0 to 10. If there is still some charge on it, continue to tap through the points, repeating those words and the feelings that come with them. Review the movie again. When you get to the point where you can retell it through that key point without experiencing any emotional charge, keep moving forward, telling the rest of the story, stopping at any emotionally charged moments to do more tapping, as you did above. When you can tell the whole story without any charge, you know you've cleared it.

Unpeeling the Layers of Emotional Events

Emotional events are different from physical ones; they affect us first and foremost on an emotional level, not a physical level. They often encompass longer periods of time and include multiple layers of emotion—all of which need to be released for full pain relief.

Just recently Debbie had learned that her husband's employer was relocating him to Kentucky. The news had come suddenly and unexpectedly, and Debbie was feeling incredibly overwhelmed. It had taken her years to get their special-needs daughter settled into a residential school where they lived in California. The thought of moving her to a new school was more than she could handle. To make matters worse, the chronic pain in Debbie's hip and right hand had become relentless. "I feel like I'm drowning in my emotions," she shared, fighting back tears as she spoke.

To begin quieting the growing sense of panic Debbie was experiencing, we began with several rounds of general tapping to release her feelings of being over-whelmed about her husband's recent news. Once she was feeling a bit more re-laxed, I asked her to tell the story of when her pain had started. It was a few years earlier, she explained, when she'd put their daughter into a residential school. "But the guilt has been there since I found out I was pregnant," she added. I asked her to tell the story of her pregnancy while tapping through the points. "I was 29. I didn't want to be pregnant. I didn't want to be a mom," she said through sobs.

At one point during the pregnancy, she'd been put on bed rest. During that time, her dad stayed with her. He was a "New Age thinker" who had always taught her that beliefs create reality. Thinking he had come to help her, Debbie had been shocked when her dad had accused her of sabotaging her pregnancy. "The child wants to abort itself because you don't want her, so you need to tell her that you want her and love her," he told her. Overwhelmed by guilt about not wanting to be pregnant, Debbie was devastated by her dad's comment. Years had passed since then, of course. "I've grown tremendously since becoming a mother," she explained. "But I also think that comment is what prompted me to believe that I had to stop being Debbie and start being nothing but a mom on a quest."

So often, when traumatic events occur, we try to convince ourselves that the lessons we learned and wisdom we gained mean that we've moved on. While on some levels we may have moved on, as we've seen, the emotions we felt as a result of the trauma can get stuck in the body. Until we fully release those emotions, the body will continue to create chronic pain. The pain is the body's way of getting our attention, telling us that something has gotten stuck. Until we fully process those emotions, we often can't end the pain.

To continue peeling back the layers of her emotional event, I then asked Debbie where she felt guilt in her body. "In the pit of my stomach, I feel like I want to throw up. And physically, it's like I'm being choked. I can't breathe," she said. We did some tapping on all the guilt in her body. Knowing that we hadn't yet gotten to the deeper layers of her pain, I then asked what, specifically, she felt guilty about. She hesitated. "Whenever I try to do anything, even get a new job, I end up having to quit because of my daughter. It's so frustrating! Something always happens, and I can never do anything for myself. I don't know how to do both—be a mom *and* be Debbie," she said. I led her through some tapping on the anger and rage she felt about not being able to do anything for herself. As we were tapping, she stopped and said, "Wow, I really wouldn't have guessed that it was anger. I really thought it was guilt."

As conscious and self-aware individuals, many of us have invested time and energy into our own personal development. During that process, we naturally begin to "diagnose" our own emotional state. Debbie's self-diagnosis had been guilt about her daughter. While that guilt is important and does need attention, beneath it were much stronger emotions—Debbie's anger and rage at not being able to be anything other than a mom.

When you're tapping on your own story, it's helpful to look at it as a process, almost like a maze that can always take a different or deeper turn. So when you're probing into your own emotions, try to keep an open mind by continuing to ask yourself questions. When you connect with an emotion, the way Debbie had connected with her guilt, you first need to notice that emotion and tap on it. At the same time, however, you want to allow yourself to stay curious, to wonder, *What other emotions am I feeling? What might be underneath that emotion?*

As Debbie and I tapped on her anger, she began to share more insights into other emotions she was feeling. "Feeling anger is the most selfish thing I could possibly feel," she said. "And realizing that I'm angry makes me feel even more guilt. Being a mom is *the* most important thing. How could I feel that way?"

As Debbie and I continued to tap on her anger and rage, I added in phrases like "It's safe to feel this anger and rage." I then asked her to fill in the blank in the sentence "I feel angry because _____" while tapping through the points. For several minutes she talked nonstop, for the first time voicing her anger about being a mom and about failing to realize her dream of starting her own business. "I'm angry because when my daughter came, I had all these grandiose dreams, but I stayed with her. I wasn't a princess; I was just a pauper," she said.

"I know I'm a great mom, but I'm angry because who I thought I was and who I am are two totally different things. I'm angry at myself because everything I'm saying is the most selfish thing I could ever say," she sobbed.

Letting Ourselves Feel "Bad" Emotions

Most of us have been taught to fight our own emotions because we're not "supposed to" feel certain emotions. We've also been taught that certain emotions aren't appropriate in certain circumstances. Unfortunately, when we deny our negative emotions, they often grow stronger. When we accept them, however, we're able to release them. That's why we say, "I deeply and completely love and accept myself" in the setup statement, to train our brains to notice and accept all of our emotions so that we can then release them.

When we paused, I asked Debbie to check in with her pain. Her hip had gone from an 8 out of 10 to a 4 out of 10. I then asked her what emotion was in her hip. "Sadness," she replied. We did some tapping on that. I kept asking her that same question over and over again as we tapped. After several minutes of tapping and talking, she said that she felt fear in her hip. "I'm scared to know who I am without my daughter . . . I want to live a vibrant life, not some mundane existence, but I'm scared to start my business. I'm scared of not being enough, even though I know I have a lot to offer," she added.

As Debbie and I continued tapping on the emotions in her hip, she began to see how conflicted she was feeling. Her chronic pain was allowing her to avoid her fear by keeping her stuck in her current life. But another part of her desperately wanted out of her current life. More than anything, she wanted to be Debbie again, while also being a mom. She needed to figure out how to do both, and that was scary. Every time she'd tried to do that, something had happened that had made it feel impossible. She was afraid of being disappointed yet again.

ASK YOURSELF: Have you diagnosed your own emotional state? If so, could there be other layers you haven't yet explored?

After several more rounds of tapping on her fear and pain and her desire to move forward in her life, I checked in with Debbie about her pain, which had gone down to a 1 out of 10. "I feel like I just got a massage," she shared in a much more relaxed tone of voice. "Okay, so now that you see the kind of pain relief you can get in forty minutes of tapping, do you feel more comfortable tapping on your own?" I asked her. "Yes, definitely," she replied. "This feels really good."

While I would love to think that Debbie's pain is gone forever, given the complexity of her situation, she's probably going to need to tap on all the emotions that continue to surface. Over time, as she releases the stuck energy and emotions at deeper and deeper levels, her pain relief will likely be more comprehensive and longer lasting. At that point, she's also likely to find new ways to take better care of herself, to find her unique combination of ways to undo the perfect storm that created her own chronic pain.

Exploring Key Emotional Events in Your Life

Now that we've taken a closer look at emotional events, it's time to begin exploring how emotionally charged events in your life may have affected you. When we do this kind of probing into emotional events, it's important that you try to be your own detective. Try to address each layer of your emotions, one at a time, and then keep tapping on what else may come up.

Take a moment now to think about the time period when your pain began. What was happening a week before the pain started? A month? That day? And after? Tap through the points as you run the movie in your mind. So, for example, if you clearly identify that work was really stressful during that time, think back about why it was so stressful, what you did about it, how that stress affected other parts of your life, like your relationships, your body, your finances, and so on. If possible, speak your memories out loud as you tap through the points.

Your Future Self: Taking in the Positive

As you answer these questions, tap through the points as you feel, visualize, and imagine these aspects of your "Future Self":

- What will be different when this old story no longer has a sad ending?
- What will you be telling yourself about that time in your life?
- What will that mean for you to have put this in the past?
- What part of your life will you get back?

Audio Bonus: If you'd like some help using the Movie Technique on a specific event, I'll guide you through it in a free audio meditation that can be found here: thetappingsolution.com/painbookresources.

Diving Deeper

Now that we've begun to look at your story around what happened when your pain began, it's time to look at a common emotional event that keeps chronic pain entrenched: the diagnosis you may have received from one or several doctors. If you haven't received a diagnosis, feel free to skip to Chapter 6.

CHAPTER 5

TAPPING ON THE DIAGNOSIS

Sarah's fear and nervousness were quickly, very quickly, turning into irritation. She had already spent 90 minutes in the examination room waiting for the orthopedist to look at her hip. That cold, lifeless room with just a few old magazines to browse through wasn't enough to distract her from the wait, the pain, and the frustration that was building. Ever since she'd injured herself a year earlier, her hip had been in chronic pain, and that pain had prevented her from living the active life she'd always enjoyed, riding horses and taking care of the animals on her farm. After unsuccessfully trying several holistic pain-relief methods, she had relented and decided to see a specialist.

When the door to the exam room finally opened, the doctor walked in. With no apology for her long wait and barely a nod, he abruptly asked what the problem was. "It's my hip," she began, pointing to her right side. Before Sarah could say another word, the doctor grabbed her right foot and twisted it hard to one side. She winced in pain. "You need a hip replacement," he said flatly. In shock, Sarah tried to ask him questions, but every time she spoke, the doctor talked over her. After mechanically outlining the basics of a hip-replacement surgery, he promptly walked out, leaving her in that same cold room, but now even more dejected and disappointed than before.

Vickie's back pain had gotten so bad that she'd finally agreed to see a spinal surgeon. Since being diagnosed with scoliosis in her 20s, she'd tried it all—Rolfing, chiropractors, acupuncture, physical therapy—"basically anything and every-thing I could find that might allow me to avoid pills and conventional medicine," she explained. The pain had only gotten worse, however, and she had begun wondering if surgery was her only option. After the surgeon walked into the exam room without even saying hello, he blurted out that he'd seen her MRIs and the news wasn't good. He then proceeded to deliver devastating news about her future, with no offer of hope or comfort. As soon as he was done, he turned around and left the room.

These are just two of the hundreds of stories I've heard from clients who have been given a devastating diagnosis. That diagnosis, and often the terrible manner it's delivered in, can be like getting punched in the face. You're already stressed out by being at the doctor's office, and in walks the man or woman in the lab coat to deliver a diagnosis that seems larger than life, like a life sentence you can't control or avoid. Because our culture teaches us that doctors know best, and that our emotions are our own "problems," we're then left alone, scared and confused, to digest the traumatizing impact of the diagnosis.

To heal your pain, it's important to process and release the trauma of that experience. While I understand that the diagnosis may have come after your pain began, it's likely become an important layer of your relationship with your body and your pain, affecting you in subtle and not-so-subtle ways. By releasing the different pieces of that experience, you can clear stress and emotional strain that may now be contributing to your chronic pain and affecting your life experience.

How a Diagnosis Affects Your Body

In many ways, the mysterious containers we inhabit—our bodies—become a doctor's property the moment we step into the examination room. After all, doctors know things! They have big degrees that took years of study to get and a base of knowledge so intricate and complex that we couldn't possibly understand it. They have proof, too—scans and X-rays and lab reports that we can't decipher—all demonstrating cold, hard facts about what is wrong with the body that's keeping us in constant pain.

When we hear things like "You'll end up in a wheelchair," "You're going to have to learn to live with the pain," and "It's getting worse, and there's nothing we can do," many of us freeze, immediately overwhelmed by emotions such as shock and fear. In this chapter, we will begin to process those emotions, but first, let's look at how the diagnosis, and the shock, fear, and other emotions we feel, affect the body.

Imagine Marta, an otherwise healthy, active woman in her 50s. She has come to see yet another doctor, a highly respected specialist in an elite private hospital, to see why her neck and back have been causing her so much pain. Sitting in the exam room, she feels afraid but also hopeful that she will soon find a solution, with this doctor's help, and be able to resume a more normal life. When the doctor walks into the room, he offers a curt and quick hello. "I've looked at your MRI," he begins. "Your spine is deteriorating. You'll probably end up in a wheelchair. There's nothing we can do to stop it."

Hearing the doctor's words, Marta's heart begins beating quickly. She begins to perspire, and it suddenly feels hard to breathe. Her brain's alarm center, the amygdala, is on high alert. The equivalent of a five-alarm fire signal is ringing in her brain, initiating the fight-or-flight stress response we discussed earlier. Every cell in her body is soon swimming in hormones, including the stress hormone cortisol, plus adrenaline and various other chemical messengers. Her brain is preparing her body to escape from danger, even though Marta can't do anything to fend off the diagnosis her doctor just delivered to her without any hope or solace.

Marta's rational forebrain is trying to tell her amygdala that it can't be true, that she needs to stay calm and ask questions for the few remaining minutes her doctor will stay in the room with her. But it's too late. Her amygdala has long since taken over, and there's little she can do to stop her body and brain from continuing to bathe her cells in stress-related hormones.

Unfortunately, when the amygdala gets triggered and the body initiates the stress response, the body's natural health-boosting mechanisms, which are responsible for relieving pain, fighting infection, slowing aging, and so much more, get turned off. Up goes her physical pain. In rush despair, anxiety, fear, and depression. Her pain worsens. Her sleep decreases, and her metabolism slows. Her body's defense mechanisms remain shut down. Her body is now working against her, and the trauma of the diagnosis will remain with her, increasing the chances that her body will fulfill the doctor's prognosis for her future.

That's just a brief snapshot of what happens in your body when you receive a serious diagnosis. As you can see, the diagnosis itself becomes an agent of destruction, contributing to your pain and interfering with your well-being. The question is, how can we reverse this downward spiral?

Releasing the Memory of Your Diagnosis

Vickie was one of three attendees who had volunteered to come up onstage to share the stories of their diagnoses. It was the first morning of my three-day pain event, so nearly everyone in the room was still in significant pain. As she listened to Thomas, who was seated next to her, tell the story of his diagnosis, her face streamed with tears. When it was Vickie's turn to share, I asked how she was doing. "I'm emotional about my diagnosis . . . the fear of it and the fear of my future and what the men in the coats have led me to believe," she responded as the tears continued down her cheeks. "How's the pain?" I asked. "It's about an eight, in the left side of my lower back," she replied. "How are you emotionally?" I then asked. "I'm a mess," she replied.

Vickie had clearly been traumatized by her diagnosis, and crying was her body's way of trying to release the emotion and energy that had gotten stuck inside her since that day. To complete the process of releasing that stuck energy and emotion, I asked her to begin tapping through the points while telling the story of her diagnosis. "Hopefulness . . . sure it couldn't be that bad, that there was some magic cure, some magic pill . . . but then, no, the diagnosis had come too late, no magic pill, no magic cure, no magic doctor. You'll end up in a wheelchair, and maybe in your seventies, twenty years from now, you can get the surgery," she shared.

I asked her to paint the picture of that day and those moments before, during, and after the diagnosis delivery. She was sitting in an exam room, she said, filled with fear. When the surgeon walked in the room, he quickly blurted out, "You're now at a fifty-degree curve. Your spine is collapsing. You've shrunk one and a half inches. It's going to keep going in this direction. Surgery's not an alternative. At your age, it's life threatening; you don't qualify. Wait another twenty years, when you'll probably need a wheelchair, and we'll see what we can do then." He exited the room soon after, leaving Vickie alone with her distress. "What did you feel when he said that?" I asked. "Shock," she said. "The shock and surprise of the diagnosis was what hit me most . . . just the brutality of telling me that way . . . He could have softened it, done anything but tell me the way he did. He didn't give me any hope at all."

To begin processing the trauma of those moments when she'd first heard the diagnosis, I led Vickie through several rounds of tapping on the shock and fear she had felt that day, as well as the brutality she had experienced from her doctor.

We also tapped on her feeling of hopelessness, finishing with, "But maybe there is a sliver of hope . . . that's all I need to get started . . . so I can relax . . . and find a way to heal." After completing several rounds, I asked her how she was feeling. "Calmer, and I feel a little more positive about moving forward," she replied. Wanting to test the strength of her new positive belief, I quickly countered, "But he said there's no hope." She nodded. "He did," she responded calmly, "but it's up to me to find the hope. And I know I will. If I'd believed him, I wouldn't have come here." The audience broke out in a big round of applause. Vickie smiled, nodding her head in determination.

ASK YOURSELF: How do you feel when you go see the doctor? Other than your diagnosis, which we'll tap on shortly, have certain other doctor visits left you feeling emotionally traumatized or upset? If so, tell the story of those visits while tapping through the points.

By the end of our tapping session onstage, Vickie's low back pain had gone from an 8 out of 10 to a 5 out of 10. And as we've already seen, thanks to the "sliver of hope" she gained during these rounds of tapping with me onstage, during a Q & A call with me several weeks after the event, she got her pain down to a 0. By releasing the trauma of her diagnosis and tapping through the tremendous stress she was feeling, she finally quieted down her amygdala's high-alert signals, and her pain went away.

I believe it's important to note here an added benefit beyond the pain going away. Calming the amygdala increases clarity, creativity, and potential for new solutions. Have you ever noticed that you have your best ideas in the shower? Or while you're walking or doing a hobby you love, like cooking or gardening? When your body and brain are more relaxed—when your amygdala's alarm system has been quieted down—you feel better emotionally, which for Vickie meant feeling more hopeful. In that more relaxed state, you're also more creative, which makes you more able to come up with better solutions. When you're relaxed, you're also likely to make better decisions. The more time you can spend in that relaxed state, the more creative you will be, and that creativity will make your life feel better and flow more smoothly.

With that goal of emotional release and relaxation in mind, let's take a look at your own diagnosis.

Releasing the Memory of Your Diagnosis

To begin exploring how your memory of the diagnosis has affected you and your body, you'll first need to record your memories in your journal. With your journal and a pen or pencil close by, think back on the event. If you don't remember many details, begin tapping through the points while focusing on anything you do remember.

- What day, month, and season was it?
- What did the doctor's office look like?
- Were you in an office or an examining room?
- What were you wearing?
- Were you alone or with someone?
- Did you have to wait for a long time?

What did the doctor say to you? Run your memories of that event through your mind, like a movie. Write down as many details as you remember, including smells, sounds, and colors.

Now let's do some tapping on that event. Rate the intensity of your memory on a scale of 0 to 10. Also, make a note of where your pain is on a scale of 0 to 10 when you're recalling this memory.

Next, tell the story of your diagnosis, out loud if possible, while tapping through the points. If there are words the doctor said to you that still carry an emotional charge, when you get to that point in the story, say those words out loud repeatedly as you tap through the points until the words no longer hold an emotional charge for you.

It might sound like this:

Eyebrow: They asked me to get dressed and then took me into the doctor's office . . .

Side of Eye: I remember sitting there looking around his office, looking at the things on his desk, the pictures on the wall.

Under Eye: I remember feeling cold and out of my body . . .

Under Nose: When he walked in he sat down and just said—you have spinal stenosis . . .

Chin: Just like that.

Collarbone: You have spinal stenosis.

Under Arm: No warning—just flat out . . .

Top of Head: And I remember sitting there thinking, *This can't be real . . .*

Notice that when he said, "You have spinal stenosis," shock and anger come up. Stop there and go through the points, using his words and stating your emotions.

Eyebrow: You have spinal stenosis.

Side of Eye: You have spinal stenosis.

Under Eye: There's this huge pit in my stomach . . .

Under Nose: It's like I'm out of my body.

Chin: Those words . . .

Collarbone: You have spinal stenosis . . .

Under Arm: I can't believe he just dumped that on me . . .

Top of Head: As if it were nothing.

Eyebrow: You have spinal stenosis.

Side of Eye: I'm so angry with him.

Under Eye: He could have been softer.

Under Nose: He didn't have to be so cold.

Chin: What the heck . . .

Collarbone: Who does that . . .

Under Arm: What a jerk!

Top of Head: What a jerk!

Continue tapping through the points as you give voice to all the emotions coming up as you recall hearing the diagnosis. Don't be surprised if you find yourself getting in touch with different emotions, such as sadness, as you do this process. It's all part of peeling back the layers.

When you're ready, stop and check in with yourself on the intensity of the memory and/or words the doctor said, as well as the intensity of your pain. Give each one a number, on a scale of 0 to 10. Keep tapping through the memories and/or words until the intensity is a 3 or lower. When you're ready, check in on your pain, and make a note in your journal of any shifts you experienced in your pain while tapping on the memory of your diagnosis.

Emotional Trauma of the Diagnosis

When we're looking at the emotional impact of a diagnosis, we sometimes discover multiple layers of emotion, so, for instance, anger toward a doctor may be masking even deeper emotions we need to process and clear in order to get pain relief.

As she told the story of her doctor twisting her foot and announcing that she needed a hip replacement, Sarah began talking faster and faster. While her story was focused on the logistics of that day, her speech and body language clearly suggested that she was experiencing a high level of emotion. Before she could continue, I stopped her. "I'm going to ask you to pause here," I said. "As you talk about this, how are you feeling?" Without hesitation, she replied, "I'm angry."

Many of you have told and retold the story of your diagnosis. Instead of simply repeating the story the way you always have, your goal here is to tell the story with a new awareness. It's important to notice not just what happened, how you were treated, and what was said and done, but also how you were feeling when it happened and how you feel when you recall that memory. As you tap through your own diagnosis, try to notice the emotions and energy behind your memories. As we've seen, they can get lodged in the body and then contribute to pain.

"Tell me about the anger," I said to Sarah next.

"I was insulted. I was outraged. I felt he was so arrogant, and he shut me down every time I asked him a question. He assumed I'd get a second opinion, so he was done with me right away. He spent less than ten minutes with me and couldn't wait to get out of the room. I just wanted to reach out and strangle him." We did several rounds of tapping on her diagnosis, focusing on her anger and outrage at the doctor and her desire to strangle him.

When we were done, I asked how she was feeling. "My anger shifted," she replied, "from anger at him to anger at my hip and my body for not healing it. I feel like my body has betrayed me. I've always held a strong belief that the body can heal itself and has amazing abilities. While my hip is a lot better than it was, I still can't do the one thing that I love, which is riding my horse, and there's no hope other than this hip replacement, so I feel like I'm somehow failing . . . My stupid hip, I'm just so mad at it."

I asked her where she feels that anger at her body and her hip. "In my neck, my jaw clenches," she answered. We then did several rounds of tapping on her anger at her hip and her body. Afterward, I asked her how she was feeling about her hip. "I'm not angry at it anymore," she said. "It's still a stupid hip," I said. "It's still a stupid hip," she agreed, "and I still don't trust it, but I'm not angry at it."

• •

Many of you have told and retold the story of your diagnosis. Instead of simply repeating the story the way you always have, your goal here is to tell the story with a new awareness. It's important to notice not just what happened, how you were treated, and what was said and done, but also how you were feeling when it happened and how you feel when you recall that memory.

• •

Once Sarah had been able to clear her anger at her hip, she could connect with another layer of her experience—mistrust.

Exploring the Emotions Around Your Diagnosis

To begin, get your journal and a pen or pencil. When you're ready, ask yourself, *How did I feel before seeing the doctor? While he or she was speaking? Afterward? How do I feel now, as I remember it?* Write down the different emotions you experienced at different points in the event—hope, fear, shock, disbelief, anger, loneliness, hopelessness, and so on.

Next, look at your list and pick the emotion that feels most intense for you right now. Give it a number from 0 to 10, and give your pain a separate number from 0 to 10. Now, let's do some tapping! We'll use anger as an example, but feel free to replace it with your own emotion.

Karate Chop: Even though I have so much anger about my diagnosis, I deeply and completely love and accept myself.

Karate Chop: Even though I have all this anger at the doctor and the way he treated me, I choose to accept myself now.

Karate Chop: Even though I'm angry at this diagnosis and how powerless it makes me feel, I still accept myself.

Eyebrow: I have so much anger about this . . .

Side of Eye: I'm angry that this has happened to me.

Under Eye: I'm angry at him for how he treated me . . .

Under Nose: I'm mad at this diagnosis.

Chin: I'm mad at the doctor.

Collarbone: He took away my hope.

Under Arm: He took away my future.

Top of Head: I am so angry right now . . .

Eyebrow: All this anger in my body . . .

Side of Eye: All this anger with my body . . .

Under Eye: I'm angry and I don't know what to do now.

Under Nose: I'm mad this is happening!

Chin: I'm angry and I feel helpless.

Collarbone: How dare they treat me that way . . .

Under Arm: How dare they take my hope . . .

Top of Head: I won't let them!

Check in with yourself. How do you feel emotionally? Has your physical pain shifted? Keep tapping on the "negative" until your emotional intensity is a 5 or lower and then switch to some positive rounds. Remember, these scripts are just here for guidance and to get you started. Feel free to use your own language, speak your own truth, and so forth.

Positive Round

Eyebrow: I choose to take my power back.

Side of Eye: I choose to be hopeful.

Under Eye: I choose to be empowered.

Under Nose: I choose to let some of this anger go . . .

Chin: My body doesn't need this anger.

Collarbone: I choose to help my body be strong.

Under Arm: The more I help my body feel calm . . .

Top of Head: The more I take my power back.

When you're ready, pause your tapping to check in with yourself. Rate the intensity of your emotion(s) from 0 to 10, and give your physical pain a separate number. Continue tapping on the emotion(s) around your diagnosis until the intensity is a 3 or lower. Then rate the intensity of your pain separately and make a note of any shifts you experienced in your pain as you tapped on these emotions.

Unearthing Beliefs about What's Possible

After you've tapped on the emotions surrounding your diagnosis and pain, it's important to go even one level deeper: exploring what beliefs that these experiences may have created. Many beliefs, such as "I'll never heal," "Life is going to be hard," or "I'm not strong enough to get through this," can lead to an inability to heal.

"It's like getting back together after a bad breakup, right?" I joked with Sarah as we continued discussing her mistrust of her hip. "You're basically telling your hip, 'I don't trust you yet, but I've let go of some of the anger.'" She nodded, laughing. I asked her where she thought her mistrust was coming from.

"Every time I go to engage the muscles around my hip," she explained, "especially when I ride my horse, it will start hurting right away or soon afterward . . . Or if my horse stops to look at something or trips and jostles me in any way, I feel like I'm going to crumble in pain like a house of cards."

Hearing Sarah talk, it was clear that she had thought through these scenarios at great length. Because of her "stupid hip," she had created a belief that riding her horse, or using her hip muscles in any way, equaled pain. That belief had originated from a fall she'd experienced while riding her horse, and it had become even more ingrained since being diagnosed with severe arthritis and told she needed a hip replacement. Hearing her doctor's recommendation, she'd understood that her "stupid hip" was useless and, therefore, riding her horse was out of the question.

When we're looking at beliefs, it's important to remember that your body, including your amygdala, is always trying to keep you safe. If you have a belief that your diagnosis makes you unable to do certain activities without experiencing pain, your body may try to protect you by creating pain when you attempt that activity. While it may feel like your body is betraying you by creating that pain, in fact, it is only trying to guard you against danger.

As we began tapping on her mistrust of her hip, we both began to laugh. The words we were saying sounded so much like a lovers' spat that I said so and asked her to take us through her lovers' spat with her hip while tapping on the points.

"You have to do what I tell you to," she began.

"Well, that's a good start to a relationship," I joked.

Laughing, she continued: "I'm in charge. I tell you what to do, and you do it happily, without any complaints . . . This is a dictatorship," Sarah added. Now the audience was laughing along.

"I want to be able to do what I want to do, and not hurt before, during, or after," she said.

"Okay, you've had your turn," I said. "Now let's give your hip a chance to talk."

In case you're thinking I've gone off the deep end, asking her hip to "talk," keep in mind that exercises like this can be really powerful. We live in a culture that teaches us to disassociate from our bodies, a culture that has led us to believe that a doctor you've never met understands what's going on in your own body better than you do. While that may be partially true at times, it's not always. Because Western medicine views the human body as a purely physical collection of cells, nerves, muscles, and bones that's separate from thoughts and emotions, we're often unconsciously programmed to ignore or mistrust the body's signals. And that programming can cause us to unconsciously override what the body wants and needs in order to meet cultural standards and expectations. When we tap while tuning in to the specific body part that was diagnosed, however, we can begin to reverse that cultural programming and hear what the body is trying to tell us.

"So, what does your hip want to say?" I asked Sarah a second time.

"It wants to say, 'Yes, ma'am,'" she said as the entire audience once again broke out in laughter.

"I know that's what you want your hip to say, but let's give it a chance to say what it wants to tell you," I suggested.

She laughed, took a deep breath, and continued tapping. "I do the best I can . . . sometimes I just need a break . . . we've been through a lot over the years . . . we needed to make some changes . . . a lot of good has come from this . . . we've grown . . . we've learned . . . that nothing's impossible."

As we kept tapping, I asked her how she was feeling. "I feel at peace with my hip; it's not my enemy," she shared. "I can't force it to heal. We need to work together."

I looked out at the audience. "Is that a better relationship than the one she started with?" I joked as everyone laughed.

Eager to test our progress, I checked in with Sarah on her pain. It's really important to keep doing this as you tap, to see if you still feel angry or sad or hopeless or whatever you were feeling before you tapped on your diagnosis, and then see whether it affects your pain.

"My pain is better," she shared, "but it's still there if I move my hip. It's less, though, and now it has no trigger. There's no story behind it now. Before, when I would think about it, there was a story I would get all worked up over. Now it's just pain."

By the end of our tapping together onstage, the story of her diagnosis had lost its emotional hold over her. She could think about her doctor, her hip, and her body without feeling tormented by anger or mistrust or any other negative emotions. Huge progress! Having cleared so much negative emotion, she could continue to tap through her belief that riding her horse would cause her pain. Whether she discovers additional beliefs that need attention, or is able to get pain relief by fully clearing that belief, by releasing all that energy during our tapping, she's supporting her body's ability to heal and relieve pain.

ASK YOURSELF: Does pain relief seem impossible because of your pain and your diagnosis? Tap on it, and then keep tapping on it more. Beliefs like these can become ingrained, and sometimes they take time to clear.

So far we've looked at how emotions and beliefs around your diagnosis can contribute to pain and how we begin to clear them. What we haven't yet seen is how releasing limiting beliefs creates new possibilities in our lives.

New Beliefs, New Possibilities

When Patricia first woke up in the ER, she had no idea what had happened. The medical staff surrounding her quickly informed her that she'd broken her back and couldn't walk. She required emergency surgery to save her bowels, legs, and bladder. Recalling that traumatic moment, she added, "The pain took my breath away."

Patricia had been severely injured in a boating accident that had happened during a first date. Her date had been driving his boat very fast, and after falling down hard at a bad angle, she had shattered her L1, one of the large lumbar vertebrae of the lower back. Hours later, Patricia's lower back had been surgically reconstructed and now contained four titanium rods and eight sets of screws and bolts, which would keep her spine intact from that point onward. While the surgery had been deemed successful, Patricia was devastated to learn from her doctors that she would probably always have pain and would be unable to resume the physically active life she'd always enjoyed.

Her doctors' dire prognosis had destroyed Patricia's vision of her future, as well as her self-image as an independent, active, positive person. In the months after the surgery, she was constantly aware of a dead weight in her lower back, almost like a brick had been strapped to it. Her pain was unrelenting, and her days were consumed by thoughts of what she could and couldn't do because of her injury. In addition to taking pain medicine throughout her days, she had been forced to take sleep medicine most nights.

Struggling with her new reality, Patricia applied for the four-day retreat I hosted in 2007, which was later made into the movie *The Tapping Solution*. During the retreat, Patricia worked with the group as well as with individual tapping coaches, such as my friend Rick Wilkes, on the different layers of her pain, including training Patricia's brain to accept the rods, screws, and bolts in her back as the "new normal." The brain can be very effective at rejecting objects in the body that it doesn't recognize, so it was important to create a new belief that her surgically reconstructed lower back could be a healthy part of her body, rather than a constant reminder of trauma and injury.

By the end of the retreat, Patricia's pain decreased dramatically, and then it disappeared completely soon after. Even more important, she wasn't constantly aware of her back and didn't feel that same heaviness she had throughout the previous many months. Using tapping to create new beliefs about herself, her back, and her injury, she no longer needed to identify herself as an injured person. This created an entirely new set of possibilities for her future.

Six months after the retreat, Patricia was still using tapping on a regular basis to process her emotions and transform other beliefs. She was also hiking, doing yoga, traveling, and more. Her back pain was gone, and she no longer needed medication for pain relief or sleep. She said that she rarely thought about her back or her injury now. In fact, during a recent trip, a friend had repeatedly offered to carry Patricia's luggage. Patricia couldn't figure out why, until finally she realized that it was because of her injury. "I don't think about my back most of the time," she explained. "It's almost like it never happened."

Even with rods, screws, and bolts permanently implanted in her back, and zero hope from her doctors for returning to an active life, she was able to use tapping to create a completely new set of beliefs for herself and then turn her new positive beliefs into new possibilities in her life. Because she continued to use tapping regularly, even after her physical pain and discomfort went away, her life changed on every level. Emotionally, she said she felt more positive and calmer on a daily basis, and by keeping her body in a more relaxed state, she's giving her body constant support for healing and also preventing her pain and discomfort from returning. I checked in with Patricia recently, to see how she was doing, and a full seven years after the retreat, she was pain-free. What a transformation!

Patricia's story is a powerful example of how this process can transform your world, inside and out, regardless of how serious your diagnosis may be.

Now that we've seen what's possible when we tap through limiting beliefs around a diagnosis, let's take a look at some of the limiting beliefs you may have around your own diagnosis.

Limiting Beliefs Around a Diagnosis

As we saw with Patricia, a diagnosis can quickly become an integral part of who you are and what you're capable of doing. When you're in that mind-set, it's easy to create limiting beliefs that hold you back. To get started, let's look at some of the most common limiting beliefs related to diagnoses that I've seen in clients:

• My condition is really serious. I don't think tapping can help.

- My doctor said the pain will probably never go away.

- Every time I exercise or make this or that movement, it hurts. The doctor said not to do anything that causes pain.

- My doctor said I can't <fill in the blank> because of my condition, so there's not much I can do to change that.

- The doctor said my condition will only get worse with time.

- I saw it on an X-ray/MRI. The reality is, I just have a bad <knee/back/hip/etc.>.

- It's a physical condition, not one related to my emotions!

- My condition is degenerative, so all I can do is manage the pain and discomfort as my body continues to deteriorate.

- I don't have many options. My doctor said there was no cure.

This list could go on and on, but you get the picture.

When we're looking at beliefs around a diagnosis, we also need to consider the flip side, which is what you believe about healing your body and getting pain relief. For instance, someone who believes that his or her condition is too serious for tapping to help probably also believes on some level that his or her chronic pain will never go away. Likewise, someone who believes that his condition is getting worse every day may also believe that healing and total pain relief are not realistic goals.

To give you a clearer sense of limiting beliefs around healing and pain relief, here are some of the most common ones I've seen in clients:

- My pain will probably never go away. My doctor told me that.

- My pain goes away for a few hours at a time here and there, but it always comes back. It's from a degenerative physical condition, so there's not much I can do.

- I have to be perfect to get pain relief and heal this disease/condition in my body.

- I have to be completely stress-free to get pain relief and heal this disease/condition in my body.

These kinds of limiting beliefs can get buried in our minds, so they're not always conscious thoughts or things we typically say out loud. As we've seen, they often feel more like truths, underlying assumptions that shape how we think, what makes sense to us, and what seems possible and impossible.

To begin identifying some of your limiting beliefs around your diagnosis, next we'll do a journaling and tapping exercise. Later in this book, we'll be taking a deeper look at other beliefs you may have about your body and your pain, so for now, we'll focus only on limiting beliefs that are related to your diagnosis.

Exploring Your Beliefs about Your Diagnosis

Before we begin, take a moment to get your journal and a pen or pencil. When you're ready, take a deep breath and tap through the points while asking yourself, *What do I believe to be true about my pain and my body because of my diagnosis? What is and isn't possible for me because of my diagnosis?*

Continue asking yourself these questions while tapping through the points. When you've gotten some answers, write them all down in your journal. When you're done, read through your list. Now let's do some general tapping on them:

Karate Chop: Even though I have these beliefs about this diagnosis, I deeply and completely accept myself and I'm open to a new way of seeing this.

Karate Chop: Even though everyone knows the facts about this pain, about this diagnosis—who am I to be different?—I still accept myself now and I'm open to a new way of seeing this.

Karate Chop: Even though it would take a miracle to heal my pain/my diagnosis, and miracles don't happen for me, I choose to accept myself and I'm open to a new way of seeing this.

Eyebrow: I don't believe I will be pain-free.

Side of Eye: They don't think it's possible.

Under Eye: I may get some relief . . .

Under Nose: But I expect the pain to come back.

Chin: I have this conviction . . .

Collarbone: That it's not possible for me to be pain-free.

Under Arm: I would have to make lots of changes in my life . . .

Top of Head: And I don't think it would matter.

Eyebrow: I probably wouldn't stick with it.

Side of Eye: Besides, it's not possible to be pain-free.

Under Eye: I want to believe it could be possible . . .

Under Nose: Although I'm not there yet.

Chin: I want to believe it's possible . . .

Collarbone: But I don't want to be disappointed.

Under Arm: I don't want to let others down.

Top of Head: It seems safer to be skeptical.

Check in with yourself. How do you feel emotionally? Has your physical pain shifted? Keep tapping on the "negative" until your emotional intensity is a 5 or lower and then switch to some positive rounds. As always, use language that reflects your own truth.

Positive Round

Eyebrow: What if it were possible to be pain-free . . .

Side of Eye: What if I could change this belief . . .

Under Eye: I would like to believe it's possible . . .

Under Nose: Maybe it is possible . . .

Chin: I want to be open to it being possible.

Collarbone: I'm ready to experience new possibilities.

Under Arm: I'm choosing to accept there could be new possibilities.

Top of Head: I'm open to new possibilities with this pain.

Next, choose one belief that feels especially true. Because beliefs are so ingrained in how we think, to really transform them, it's a good idea to focus on one at a time. Once you've chosen the belief you want to start tapping on, ask yourself how true it feels on a scale of 0 to 10, and also make a note of how intense your pain is when you think about it. Then start tapping, beginning with the following setup statement: "Even though I have this belief that <your belief here>, I deeply and completely love and accept myself."

Continue tapping through the points until you feel a shift or identify another layer. Check in on how true the original belief feels when you're done, and also whether your pain has shifted. Make notes of any changes you experienced in your journal.

Beliefs often take the longest to transform because they're the roots of your emotions and your thinking, so don't worry if you later find that this belief is still with you. Clearing limiting beliefs can take time, and you don't necessarily need to clear all of them to get the pain relief you desire. Remember also to stop and appreciate every shift you experience, in your pain, your emotions, and your beliefs, as well as in your mood and overall sense of well-being.

Up to this point in this process, we've looked at two specific events within your larger story—what was happening when your pain first began and your diagnosis. Next we'll step back and take a broader look at how your emotions may be contributing to your pain and how to release them in a healthy and lasting way.

Your Future Self

As you answer these questions, tap through the points as you feel, visualize, and imagine these aspects of your "Future Self":

- What do you believe about possibilities?

- What does hope look like?

- What does determination look like?

Audio Bonus: If you want some help tapping on the diagnosis, join me in a free audio tapping meditation here: thetappingsolution.com/painbookresources.

CHAPTER 6

EXPRESSING AND CLEARING EMOTIONS

Anya sat down at her computer, hoping to get some work done in spite of the pain in her lower back. Scrolling through her e-mail in-box, she noticed an e-mail from me, opened it, and clicked on the link inside to watch a video interview I'd done with Wayne Dyer. In the video, Wayne and I were discussing the importance of releasing anger in order to experience forgiveness. While watching the video, Anya was overcome by her anger toward her husband about their divorce. She immediately began tapping along with the video, allowing herself to feel the full force of her anger as she did. By the end of the video, Anya felt calmer. Much to her surprise, her back pain had also vanished!

Excited about her results, she wrote me an e-mail thanking me for sharing the video. In it she explained that she wasn't surprised that her low back pain had been connected to her anger about the divorce. Before tapping along with the video, however, she had assumed her pain was connected to an injury, rather than to her emotions.

It's the story I hear all the time. On some level we know how powerful our emotions are, and how intimately connected they are to the state of the physical body. We often imply that understanding when we say things like "I'm so upset, I feel sick," "You make me sick to my stomach," and "My heart aches." But when we're suffering from pain that won't go away, we don't stop to ask ourselves whether our emotions could be causing it. Instead, we focus our attention on our physical anatomy as the primary source of pain.

To many people, it makes perfect sense that emotions associated with their pain can prolong it, but it's often harder for them to recognize the power of emotions that aren't directly associated with their pain, injury, or diagnosis. But as you probably understand by now, our emotions and anatomy are part of the same intricately interconnected system. Until we process and release the deeper emotions that have gotten stuck in the body, we can't heal chronic pain.

To understand why this is, let's step back and take a look at how the primitive parts of the brain handle different emotions, what we believe about emotions, and how those beliefs may impact the body.

. . . .

Our emotions and anatomy are part of the same intricately interconnected system. Until we process and release the deeper emotions that have gotten stuck in the body, we can't heal chronic pain.

. . . .

Accessing Deeper Emotions

When I first ask clients what emotions they're experiencing, they often say they feel "frustrated," "stressed," or "overwhelmed." As we dig into their stories, many are surprised to discover repressed emotions they weren't aware they had buried, like rage, anger, fear, and sadness. Once they're able to feel and release these deeper emotions through tapping, they often experience the pain relief they're seeking.

So why is it so challenging for us to connect with the deeper emotions that are contributing to chronic pain?

Earlier we learned about the brain's ingrained negativity bias and how the brain is programmed to feel fear more readily. This same desire for protection by the unconscious mind also interferes with our ability to access deeper emotions.

As just one example, the primitive, unconscious mind, which includes the amygdala, might react to the emotion of loneliness the same way you would consciously react to the sound of footsteps in an abandoned alley. It sees loneliness as an immediate threat, something to be afraid of, rather than an emotion it can process and release without harm. As a result, it tries to protect you from that loneliness by preventing your conscious mind from accessing it, similar to the way you might run away from footsteps in an abandoned alley in order to escape whoever might be pursuing you.

From a cultural standpoint, I also think we receive so much conflicting information about emotions that we don't know how to face them. As children, we're told we shouldn't be angry; we get punished for having tantrums or expressing our frustration, so we learn to swallow those emotions. Instead of expressing our anger in a healthy way by standing up for ourselves and saying how we feel, we either shut down our anger or let it erupt. Both of these choices often lead to negative consequences—emotional pain and unwanted disruptions in our lives and relationships. Starting at a young age, "being emotional" begins to seem dangerous, and emotions such as anger, sadness, guilt, and shame begin to seem "bad."

As adults, the confusion often continues. We see information about the law of attraction or positive thinking, all important stuff, but we misinterpret it to mean we should never feel negative emotions, and then we bury them even further! The question is, then, if we can't avoid feeling negative emotions, what do we do with them?

Expressing "Bad" Emotions

Science has shown that, as far as the body is concerned, there is no such thing as a "bad" emotion. The only emotions that do any actual harm to the body are the ones we repress. Let me repeat that, because it's really important: all of our emotions are healthy and normal, including anger, sadness, rage, fear, and more, as long as we let ourselves feel them and then let them go. The only emotions that the body sees as threatening are the ones we don't express fully.

When we're looking to relieve chronic pain, one of the most important changes we can make is to let ourselves feel and express more of our emotions when we're tapping. To begin that process, we first need to retrain our brains to know that it's safe to express emotions, especially negative ones. Using tapping, we can let the unconscious mind know that we won't be hurt or harmed if we "let it all out."

Feeling Safe Expressing Emotions

It was the first session on the first day of my pain-relief event, and three volunteers from the audience had just joined me onstage. Once they were settled in their seats, I asked them to share their stories. Thomas went first. "I was diagnosed with rheumatoid arthritis in 2003. It was crippling, and they put me on medication to manage the deterioration in the joints, but it's . . . frustrating. They put me on several medications, and they keep prescribing them, but they don't really help with the pain," he shared, wincing as he spoke. "The pills are a meal unto themselves." He smiled. Thomas's pain was in several places—his chest, shoulders, hips, knees, wrists, and feet. The worst pain was in his wrist, he shared, which was an 8 out of 10.

· ·

When we're looking to relieve chronic pain, one of the most important changes we can make is to let ourselves feel and express more of our emotions when we're tapping.

· ·

When I asked him what thoughts and emotions came up when he thought about his diagnosis, he abruptly looked down again. His face darkened as he swallowed several times. "Wanting to numb up," he replied after several seconds of silence. "I'm always trying to distance myself from the emotions," he added, pausing again before continuing. "The year that diagnosis happened, I was kidnapped and tortured by some white supremacists." He paused, nodded, and looked up at me for the first time since beginning to share his story. His face was tight. Looking into his eyes, I could see that he had reached his limit and couldn't say any more.

Like many trauma survivors, Thomas had survived the event but had never been given the opportunity to process the emotions behind it. Every time he alluded to that trauma, I could see him fighting back tears and swallowing repeatedly, trying so hard to push away the huge waves of emotion that were buried inside him. He just couldn't let himself go there, though. The emotional pain was too great.

I led him through several rounds of tapping, beginning with "Even though I want to numb this emotion . . . it's not safe to feel it . . . I deeply and completely love and accept myself." As Thomas was tapping with me, he went silent and stopped tapping as I was saying, "I deeply and completely love and accept myself." Noticing his silence, I began another round with "Even though I can't feel this . . . it's too scary . . . It's too big . . . I just don't want to go there, I deeply and completely love and accept myself." When we got to "I deeply and completely love and accept myself," Thomas shook his head no, and said, "I can't." I nodded, and began again with "Even though I can't go there, I can't love myself, I can't even say it, I choose to relax now." Thomas repeated the entire setup statement, and we continued tapping on wanting not to feel his emotions because it felt too scary, too unsafe. We ended with several rounds of tapping on "I can't accept myself with it . . . I don't want to go there . . . and I accept myself . . . even if I don't want to go there."

Here's a possible list of different affirmations for when you can't accept yourself:

- I am willing to accept a new attitude.
- I want to be able to accept myself.
- I intend to be able to accept myself someday.
- I choose to feel calm now.
- I choose to change the way I feel about myself.
- I choose to feel calm and confident.
- I'm allowing myself to feel calm now.
- I choose to know that a divine force loves me.

In a culture that's focused on positive thinking, it can be tempting to try to force ourselves to say statements like "I deeply and completely love and accept myself," but with tapping, it's important to recognize and respect how you're actually feeling. Try to honor your emotions, no matter what they are, or how dark and negative they seem. The more you allow yourself to feel what you're feeling when you're tapping, the more quickly you'll be able to release those negative emotions and experience relief from your pain.

When we were done, I asked Thomas how he was feeling. "I actually felt my neck loosen up a bit . . . and it's easier to breathe right now . . . I had never allowed myself to feel. I come from a tribal position where I'm a leader and you're not supposed to show feelings . . . and I've never been able to voice how I'm feeling. Sometimes that made me angry because you're supposed to feel something, aren't you?" I asked him to repeat the statement "It's not safe to feel," and then asked him how true that felt. He said it was an 8 out of 10. I asked him who taught him that. "My dad," he said. "We were never allowed to cry or show any real emotion, and every time we did, he'd say, 'I'm gonna give you something to cry about.'"

Next I asked him to picture a feeling meter in his heart, with 10 being wide open, feeling all of his emotions, and 0 being feeling no emotions at all. "Where do you live in that feeling meter on an everyday basis?" I asked him. "Maybe about a six," he replied, "but when it comes to that issue, it's a zero," referring to the trauma he'd experienced. We did several more rounds of tapping, focusing on it not being safe to feel, what he'd learned from his dad, and how being a leader had prevented him from feeling. We ended with "It's not safe to feel . . . not feeling is part of who I am . . . but maybe I can feel . . . no, I can't . . . I can feel sometimes . . . but not about the big things . . . they're too big to feel . . . they're too painful to feel . . . it's too painful to accept myself . . . with all these feelings."

When we're unearthing emotions the unconscious mind never wanted us to face, it's normal to feel unsure about "going there." Again, it's important to acknowledge those feelings when you're tapping, because you can't release them until you allow yourself to feel them.

ASK YOURSELF: Are there emotions you're not allowing yourself to feel, emotions that feel too big and overpowering to experience fully? Begin tapping as you let yourself feel them.

When we were done, I asked Thomas how his pain was. He looked down at his hands and began opening and closing his fists, moving his fingers, and making circular motions with his wrists. "I kind of felt a crick in my wrist where some of my worst pain is, and I can actually move it. The pain's only a level two now," he shared. "Do you think feeling might be connected with that pain at all?" I asked. "Yeah," he said. Then he looked up at me. "Oh yeah," he said, laughing out loud.

In that small amount of time tapping, Thomas's pain had decreased dramatically. More important, though, he'd gone from a man who was emotionally shut down and unavailable to a guy who seemed open and friendly. He could even laugh at himself and genuinely enjoy the moment. Huge difference!

After our time onstage, I didn't hear from Thomas until the lunch break on the following day, which was day two of the event. When I heard his results, I asked him if he would mind sharing with the audience. Before beginning that day's post-lunch session, I gave him the microphone.

"Second day here, zero pain," he shared as the audience started clapping and howling with excitement. "I can actually move," he said as he touched his toes, made big circular motions with his arms, and bent down as his legs seesawed from left to right. "It feels awesome!" he shared with a big smile. "I went walking through the lobby, enjoying the pain-free movement. I was doing laps and people were asking if I needed something, if I was trying to get somewhere, and I was like, I'm doing my laps, people," he said, looking the happiest and most relaxed he had yet. The audience immediately broke out in simultaneous applause and laughter.

Whether or not we've experienced trauma, we all know the experience of being punished, ostracized, or isolated for expressing emotion. As a result, over time, we begin to feel afraid of expressing our own emotions. To begin retraining our brains that it's safe to feel and express emotions, rather than repress them, let's do some tapping on that now.

When you think about expressing your emotions, how unsafe does it feel? Give it a number on a scale of 0 to 10. Also give your pain its own number. Write both of these down in your journal. Now let's get started:

Karate Chop: Even though it's not safe to feel that, I can't handle it, I still choose to accept myself and these feelings.

Karate Chop: Even though these feelings will be too much for me, I choose to consider that I can handle them now.

Karate Chop: Even though I'm afraid of feeling these feelings, that's okay, because I still choose to accept me and how I feel.

Eyebrow: I don't want to feel all these feelings . . .

Side of Eye: I've always done my best to avoid feeling them.

Under Eye: I'm not supposed to be in touch with these feelings.

Under Nose: It just isn't safe to feel them.

Chin: I know I'll be overwhelmed if I feel them.

Collarbone: Nobody in my family is good with feelings.

Under Arm: There's a rule that you're not supposed to feel your feelings.

Top of Head: Strong people never feel their feelings.

Eyebrow: I'm not sure how to handle all of these feelings . . .

Side of Eye: What if I have too many of them . . .

Under Eye: I'm sure feeling these feelings will be painful.

Under Nose: It will be overwhelming.

Chin: I won't know how to protect myself from them.

Collarbone: Perhaps I don't have to do it all at once . . .

Under Arm: Maybe I can just begin to notice some of these emotions . . .

Top of Head: I could take it slow.

Eyebrow: Maybe I can handle some of my emotions . . .

Side of Eye: What if it wasn't too much . . .

Under Eye: What if I could handle it . . .

Under Nose: I choose to trust in my ability to handle anything that comes up.

Chin: I think I can handle some of my emotions . . .

Collarbone: I think I can handle some of my emotions . . .

Under Arm: I'm willing to be open to feeling these feelings.

Top of Head: I'm ready to find I can feel feelings and still be safe.

Check in with yourself, and keep tapping until the unsafe feelings you had about expressing your own emotions are a 3 or lower. Also take note of any shifts in pain that you experience.

Once you're feeling more comfortable expressing emotion, it's time to explore what emotion(s) may be buried within your chronic pain. These emotions are often not directly connected to the pain itself, but repressing them is what keeps the pain going.

What's the Emotion Behind Your Pain?

To begin, get your journal and a pen or pencil. Close your eyes, take a deep breath, and begin tapping through the points as you ask yourself: *What emotion is behind my pain? When I see, hear, and smell the story of my pain, what emotion(s) comes up?*

There is no right or wrong answer here. Just keep tapping while asking yourself these questions repeatedly. If you get an answer like anger, fear, or guilt, ask yourself how intense that emotion feels on a scale of 0 to 10. Also take note of your pain, and give it a number on a scale of 0 to 10.

Once you pinpoint an emotion, keep tapping while asking yourself a more specific question, such as: *Fear of what? Anger at whom? Guilt about what?*

When you have your answer(s), slowly open your eyes and write down the emotion(s) and the emotional intensity number, as well as any other ideas, thoughts, or impressions that came up as you were tapping.

When I did this exercise at my pain-relief event, someone raised a hand and asked what to do if nothing came up. "Oh, then we can't help you," I joked. Then, turning to the audience, I said, "There's a broken one over here." Remember, one of the primary focuses of this process is learning to love and accept yourself. If you don't get an answer, that's okay. Some parts of the process laid out in this book will resonate with you more than others, and that's okay, too.

Whether or not you get an answer, however, I urge you to complete this entire chapter. It's such a central part of this process that everyone can benefit from.

Where Does an Emotional Pain Hurt?

Emotional pain can be located in those places in the body where emotional expression was meant to happen but failed to. For instance, if you have the urge to yell at someone who made you angry, you might develop pain in the neck, throat, and jaw—the places in your body where you held back your angry scream.

Remember, we call them feelings because we *feel* them in the body, and while your mind may be good at hiding emotions, the body can't fool itself. It has no access to denial. When your body registers an emotion, there is an accompanying physical sensation.

Although there is no one way that emotions affect the body, here are some examples of how certain emotions can look and feel in the body:

- **Anxiety** is chronic fear. You may not feel the acute signs of fear because you've grown used to them and your body has adapted. Since the body can't completely adapt, though, fear may manifest as numbness, tuning out, irritability, and sleeplessness. The body can also feel restless.

- **Anger** often manifests in the body as warmth and flushed skin, tense muscles, accelerated heartbeat, clenched jaw or fists, irregular or quick breathing, and a feeling of pounding in the ears. Anger may also begin in the back between the shoulder blades and travel upward, along the back of the neck, sometimes also around the sides of the jaws.

- **Depression** feels cold and heavy. The body is lethargic and lacking in energy. The body may move slowly, rigidly, or hesitantly.

- **Fear** may express itself as a tight stomach or chest, cramps, coldness, shaking, weakness, or dizziness. Irritable Bowel Syndrome, ulcers, indigestion, and nausea are also often related to blocked fear in a person's body.

- **Frustration** is like anger but is more pent up. It may feel like your body wants to lash out but doesn't know which way to turn. Your movements and posture may become rigid. Sometimes frustration is anger combined with denial. In this case, you will experience signs of denial, such as unusually rapid speech, shrugging, averted eyes, tightened jaw muscles, and shallow breathing.

- **Guilt** is a restless feeling. You may feel confined or suffocated, with an overwhelming desire to escape. It might feel difficult to breathe, and your chest may feel tight or pressured.

- **Hostility** is like anger but requires no trigger to set it off. Instead, the body is constantly simmering, alert for the slightest excuse for full-blown rage. The body feels tight, tense, and ready for action.

- **Humiliation** is similar to fear in that your body feels weak and sometimes shaky, but instead of feeling cold, you feel a wave of heat. You may blush and notice your skin becoming warm. You might also hunch over and retract, as if you're trying to disappear.

- **Jealousy** is a complex emotion that can contain elements of fear, humiliation, and anger. The experience of jealousy in the body may vary from one person to another. You may feel the coldness, tight stomach, and pressure in your chest associated with fear . . . or you may feel the heated sensations that come with anger and humiliation. When you find yourself clearly envying someone's life, accomplishments, relationships, or possessions, pay attention to how your body feels and you will have a baseline for what jealousy feels like when you have a more subtle experience of this emotion.

- **Rage** and **hatred** are the ultimate "gut feelings," and they often manifest in the bowels.

- **Sadness** often begins in the chest and moves upward through the throat and to the eyes, where we see tears. We've all heard the expression "She's all choked up."

- **Shame** is another heated feeling, accompanied by warm skin and flushed cheeks. However, there is also a sense of inner numbness that can feel cold or empty. Like humiliation, shame can make you hunch over, as if you're trying to disappear.

The Pain–Anger Connection

Anger is one of those big emotions that can be so overpowering, it seems like more than we can handle. We get so angry, we're "boiling," so enraged, it's "blinding." Because we never learned how to express anger in a healthy way, the experience of letting it all out is often destructive, and also unsatisfying. Think about it: when was the last time you expressed anger in a way that allowed you to let go of it for good? Oftentimes, even when we try to express anger, we find that we're still angry days, weeks, even months later. So what's the point of expressing anger at all?

It's a fair question, but in my years working with clients, I've seen what John Sarno, M.D., discovered through his many years working with thousands of patients—anger is the emotion most commonly linked to chronic pain. As he explains in *The Mindbody Prescription*, it's normal for repressed anger to manifest itself as chronic pain:

> It is important for people to know that emotionally induced physical processes [like chronic pain] are normal. The reason is clear. We all suffer the stresses and strains of everyday life, particularly if we try to be conscientious and good. "Normal" people are constantly under pressure and always generating unconscious anger-rage.

Sarno's incredible work on the link between anger and chronic pain gives us a powerful foundation for healing, and when we use tapping to release anger on a deeper level, that's when the big results happen.

When I first bring up this topic, people sometimes object to the idea that they may be holding on to repressed anger. The suggestion that they may be angry feels like an accusation, almost as if I'm pointing out something that's "wrong" with them. Again, though, we need to remember that anger is a healthy, normal response to the everyday pressures we all experience. Once we're able to express and release that anger fully, the body doesn't need to use chronic pain to get our attention, so the pain goes away.

Alyssa was a great example of the anger–pain connection. As soon as she got settled onstage on the first day of my pain-relief event, I asked her how she was feeling. "Pissed off," she said in a definitive, but slightly shaky, voice. I asked her how her pain was. "The pain in my lower back is a seven out of ten, and the pain in my hands is a ten," she replied matter-of-factly.

"Why are you pissed off?" I asked her. She replied, "I fell about ten years ago and had a traumatic foot injury. As a result of that injury, I've had six surgeries on my foot, and I also developed RSD." RSD, or Reflex Sympathetic Dystrophy, also called CRPS, is a disease associated with excruciating pain that often cannot be treated successfully through conventional medicine. The pain is so severe that some refer to RSD/CRPS as the "suicide disease."

In an attempt to treat her RSD, Alyssa explained, a doctor had implanted a neurostimulator in her back, but without following the standard protocol of taking X-rays or doing an MRI beforehand. As soon as the neurostimulator was in her back, she began experiencing electrical currents throughout her body, accompanied by terrible pain in her back. When she returned to the doctor, he took an X-ray. Soon afterward, the doctor's receptionist called her and told her to go see a neurosurgeon immediately. It was urgent.

Hearing Alyssa's voice tighten as she spoke, I stopped her and asked how she was feeling. "Really, really angry," she replied. We did a round of general tapping on her anger, and then I asked her to continue. "So I ended up having to have surgery on my back," she explained as tears streamed down her face. "I ended up having my C5 and C6 [vertebrae] fused. The surgical nurse told me I'd been *this close* to being paralyzed, and if the doctor who'd put the neurotransmitter in had followed standard protocol and done an X-ray before implanting the neurotransmitter, this never would have happened. As it turns out, I'd developed degenerative disc disease as a result of my injury, so the neurotransmitter never should have been used. And I'm just so angry at the doctor who put it in."

I asked Alyssa to visualize the doctor who'd implanted the neurotransmitter. "How do you feel?" I asked. "I'd like to punch him in the nose . . . *really* hard," she said. I asked her to feel her anger and imagine what she would say if he were in front of her now. "I never had a problem with my back before the neurotransmitter," she began, "and you didn't follow standard procedure. I never had a chance to say no to the neurotransmitter because I didn't know it would cause problems."

I asked her to visualize his face. "Okay, you still want to punch him?" I asked. "Yep," she replied. "Go ahead," I said. While tapping on the under arm point with her right hand, she made a punching motion with her left arm. Immediately after, her face softened into a big smile.

One of the most powerful ways to express and release anger is to tap while imagining yourself saying and doing the things you wish you could say and do to whomever you're angry at. By giving yourself the experience of expressing your anger verbally as well as physically while tapping, you can release it from the body more easily and quickly. It's an incredibly powerful way of processing anger without causing any harm to others or to your relationships.

The benefits of this technique seemed intuitively clear to the audience. As Alyssa was making that punching motion while tapping, I noticed several people in the audience doing the same. "Okay, you want to punch, too?" I asked the audience. "Anyone who wants to punch," I said, "just watch out for your neighbors. Punch away—just keep it straight." The room filled with laughter.

"Okay, so how did he react?" I asked, returning to Alyssa. She laughed openly, sounding sincerely gratified. "It was a hard punch and he fell on the floor." While continuing to tap, I then led her through a series of repetitive visualizations. "Feel the anger in your body," I began. "Then see your doctor on the floor . . . Feel the anger in every cell of your body, and all the months and months of chronic pain . . . and then see him on the floor."

I repeated this series seven or eight times, each time detailing her experience with chronic pain more fully. I ended every repetition with "now see him on the floor," and each time Alyssa visualized her doctor knocked down by her punch, her face relaxed into a big smile. Several times, she also laughed out loud.

When we were done tapping, I asked how she was feeling. "I feel better," she said. "Okay," I said, "so the doctor's standing up now. He's pain-free, but you're not," I said, once again testing the results. "I feel better now; I really do," she said. In less than 15 minutes of tapping, the pain in her lower back had gone from a 7 out of 10 down to a 2; the pain in her hands from a 10 out of 10 down to a 4. Just as important, Alyssa had reconnected with her emotions. After releasing her anger, for the first time in months, if not years, she could laugh and smile freely without feeling weighed down by severe and relentless pain.

Anger is sometimes called the "no trespass" emotion, and while many of us have been taught that it's a "bad" emotion that we shouldn't express, it's also the emotion that helps us create healthy boundaries. When we create healthy boundaries, we're able to say no to people, activities, and commitments that aren't in our best interests.

While each person's emotional landscape is unique, when people tap through their anger, they often discover a deep sadness—for the time they've lost because of chronic pain, relationships that have been affected, dreams that have been put aside, and more. The first step, however, is always allowing ourselves to feel the anger. It can take some practice to get in touch with anger, since most of us have gotten so good at repressing it. The best way to start is by practicing feeling anger, and then tapping through it to experience total release.

Getting in Touch with Your Anger

To begin, take a deep breath and think about all the things you have to do every day, even when you're in constant pain. Think about things that make you angry, like the way your doctor delivered your diagnosis, or all the times your boss demanded extra work from you when you were in pain, or how your family or friends told you that you need to learn to deal with the pain, even though they have no idea what it's like living with chronic pain. The anger doesn't even have to be associated with your pain. Perhaps you're angry at your mother for lying to you or you're angry at your friend for constantly showing up late. Nothing is too big or small here, so if you're angry at a stranger for running into you in the grocery store without apologizing, start with that.

Once you've picked something or someone you're angry at, give your anger a number of intensity on a scale of 0 to 10. Also notice where your pain is on a scale of 0 to 10. Write both of these down in your journal. Then focus in on your anger. Really let yourself feel it. Don't worry about whether your anger is "justified" or "acceptable." Just let yourself feel its full force, and then begin tapping. If there's a story you want to tell or a memory that's just popped in your head, speak it out loud as you tap through the points. If you want to say something to someone or imagine punching, kicking, or even throwing something at someone, imagine yourself doing that as you keep tapping. This is your time to let the floodgates of your anger open, so really go for it. Like I told the audience, though, make sure you have plenty of space around you, so no one, including you, gets hurt.

When you're ready, open your eyes and check in with your anger and your pain. Give them each a number on a scale of 0 to 10. Keep tapping until the intensity of your anger is significantly lower, no higher than a 3 out of 10. Notice also if you experience any shifts in your pain as you tap through your anger. If possible, take the time to get your anger down to a zero, even when you think about the situation or person who made you so angry in the first place. It's important that you fully release your anger so you can become familiar with that experience and further train your brain that it's safe to feel anger.

When Multiple Emotions Are Behind the Pain

When we're looking at how emotions impact chronic pain, we sometimes find that multiple emotions are contributing to the pain. That was the case for John, who, three decades and four surgeries later, still had severe back pain. A veteran of the Vietnam War, he'd also suffered PTSD after returning home from war, and more recently had had three ministrokes from Agent Orange exposure all those years ago in Vietnam. For years, he'd also had severe insomnia, extreme tinnitus (ringing in his ears), and high blood pressure.

As a result of all he'd been through, John's relationships had suffered over the years as well. When I met him in 2007 at our first tapping retreat, he was married to his third wife, who described him as "grumpy" because of his constant pain. He never laughed, she shared, and his irritable moods had caused friction in their home. Their kids would come home from school each day and ask if dad was home, afraid they'd make him angry by being too loud or disrupting him in some way.

When it was John's turn to share his story during the retreat, his gentle, easy demeanor grew darker. Forty years after coming home from war, he still had vivid memories of firing missiles and laughing with other soldiers as if it were a game (a common coping mechanism soldiers use to survive war). As he told the story, he hung his head in shame and sadness for all the violent acts of war he'd been forced to commit. Watching him, you could almost feel how heavy his burden of guilt had become. He was also angry at the elected officials at the time, he shared, for having "duped" soldiers like him into committing atrocious acts for dubious reasons.

As John tapped through his war memories, he revealed that his father had whipped and beaten him repeatedly as a child. He couldn't remember a single time when his father had expressed love or affection for him. Most often, his father would beat him on the back with a large leather strap, in the exact area where he now had chronic pain. Years later, John was carrying the tremendous anger, hurt, and sadness he felt as a result of his father's physical abuse in the same spot where he'd been beaten as a child. As John tapped through memories of his father, he could feel his back pain fading away. With each memory he cleared, the pain lessened.

To clear the emotional remnants of war, John also tapped on the guilt he felt for the violent acts he'd been ordered to commit as a soldier. In hopes of repaying the debt he felt he owed the Vietnamese people, John had spent a lot of time doing charity work in Vietnam since the end of the war. Each year, he would return several times to teach and help in any way he could. Over the years, he had also become involved in helping Vietnamese families come to the United States. Whenever families weren't allowed to come, John would get severely depressed. Each time, when the process didn't work, he would feel even more guilt, as if he had personally failed them once again.

While tapping, John realized that his guilt had become a bottomless pit. Nothing he could ever do would be enough to repay the debt he felt he owed the Vietnamese people. Even being at home with his family had grown difficult over the years. Whenever he was home for several months in a row, his guilt would become so overwhelming that he would return to Vietnam to repay more of his debt. As a result, his trips to Vietnam had become longer and longer over the years, which had further weakened his relationships with his wife and children.

After he tapped through these different layers of emotion throughout the weekend, John's back pain vanished. By the last day of the retreat, he could comfortably sit cross-legged on the floor, a position he hadn't been able to get into for many years. He also shared that his guilt felt significantly less intense.

Several months after the retreat, when my team tried to follow up with John on his progress, we weren't able to speak with him because he had gone back to Vietnam to do charity work. This time, however, his trip wasn't motivated by guilt. Instead, he had gone there to teach them tapping, simply because he loves the people there. In his absence, his wife shared that he was still pain-free and that he laughs easily and often now. He had also scheduled a shorter trip to Vietnam this time so that he could come home and be with his family. "I feel like Dad is a new person. I love this new person," his daughter shared of the changes she'd seen in him since the tapping retreat.

Let's Have a Conversation with Your Body!

Before you bolt right past this exercise, I'm going to really encourage you to hear me out and give it a try. Throughout this book we've taken a look at the way the body communicates with you, creating physical pain as a way of alerting you to repressed emotional pain that has gotten stuck in your body.

Up until now that communication has been one-sided—the body talking to you through physical pain. True communication has two sides to it, a listener and a speaker, and while your body has been talking, now that you have this new awareness of the deeper meaning of your pain, it's time for you to start to listen with a new ear.

How will others react if they find out you're talking to your body? Not to worry—no one is going to cart you off to the funny farm. You can certainly explain to them why you are doing it, or you can just simply give them your best smile, knowing that you are doing what is best for you and your body and that's all that matters.

Put your hand on the area of your body where you experience the pain. You might want to start with a little icebreaker, which might sound something like:

You: Hi, knee—it's me. I know I haven't been a very good listener up till now, but I really want that to change. I want us to work together so we can feel better. Please be patient with me because I'm new to this. I would really like to know something. If there were an emotion that I was holding in this area, what would it be?

Body: Fear.

You: What is the fear about?

Body: Fear that this won't get better.

You: Thank you, body, for trusting me, for sharing with me. I'm going to do my best to be a better listener so you don't have to get my attention with all of this pain.

After you've had this discussion with your body, give the emotion you came up with a number on a scale of 0 to 10, and give your pain its own number. Write these down in your journal, and let's do some tapping. For the person above, the tapping would go like this:

Karate Chop: Even though I'm holding this fear in my knee, I accept myself and choose to feel calm now.

Karate Chop: Even though I have this fear that it will never get better, and I'm holding it in my knee, I choose to feel calm now.

Karate Chop: Even though I have this fear that things won't get better, and there's nothing I can do about it, I accept my feelings and choose to feel calm now.

Eyebrow: I'm holding my fear in my knee . . .

Side of Eye: This fear that it will always be like this . . .

Under Eye: This fear that I will lose my independence . . .

Under Nose: This fear of losing control . . .

Chin: I'm afraid of what the future will bring.

Collarbone: This fear in my knee . . .

Under Arm: I'm not sure it's possible to feel safe.

Top of Head: This fear that I'll never feel safe . . .

Eyebrow: I don't know how to relax with this fear.

Side of Eye: I need to have this fear . . .

Under Eye: I need to stay prepared . . .

Under Nose: And expect the worst.

Chin: I want to relax, but I don't know how.

Collarbone: My body wants to feel safe . . .

Under Arm: My body wants to feel calm . . .

Top of Head: But I'm not sure how to do that.

Check in with yourself and notice how you're feeling emotionally and how your pain is. Give each a number on a scale of 0 to 10. Keep tapping on the "negative" until the intensity is a 5 or lower and then switch to some positive rounds. Remember, these scripts are just here for guidance and to get you started. Feel free to use your own language, speak your own truth, and so forth.

Positive Round

Eyebrow: This pain is part of the fear.

Side of Eye: I'm finding a way to release some of the fear . . .

Under Eye: I'm finding a way to release the pain . . .

Under Nose: I'm listening to my body now.

Chin: I'm learning to release the fear.

Collarbone: My body can relax now.

Under Arm: I'm remembering how resourceful I am.

Top of Head: It's safe for my body to release this pain and fear.

Take a deep breath and check in with yourself. Keep tapping until the intensity is a 3 or lower. Also make sure to notice any shifts in your physical pain.

Expressing emotion is an incredibly powerful, important part of being human. When we use tapping to express and release repressed emotion, like John, we often experience more than pain relief. Because we can express ourselves more fully, we can often improve our relationships and make other positive changes throughout our lives.

As we continue to dig deeper, next we'll be exploring in more detail how to process and release past traumatic experiences, particularly from childhood, that can contribute to pain.

Audio Bonus: To do more tapping on allowing yourself to feel a wider range of emotions, join me in a free audio tapping meditation here: thetappingsolution .com/painbookresources.

CHAPTER 7

RELEASING EMOTIONAL RESIDUE FROM CHILDHOOD

When I first ask clients about their childhood, I can almost hear them thinking, *What does my childhood have to do with my pain?* They'd much rather tell me what's stressing them out now; they'd rather talk about their pain, about what's going wrong. Looking at the past doesn't seem necessary, and it's also often uncomfortable. However, in my years using tapping as a pain-relief tool, I've seen more dramatic, lasting results from working through unresolved childhood memories and emotions than virtually any other area of focus and work.

I should warn you, many of you may be tempted to skip this chapter. You may see words like *trauma* and *abuse* and assume it doesn't apply to you because you had a great childhood, or you've already done a lot of work processing that time of your life. I urge you to read through this chapter and do the exercise anyway. Even when we feel as if we've moved on, there's often emotional energy from childhood that's gotten stuck in the body. Even people who had great childhoods can develop chronic pain as a result of unresolved childhood experiences and emotions, sometimes simple ones that don't even seem that important at first glance. By releasing the emotional intensity of the past, the charge that it holds, you'll also enjoy more peace of mind and likely find more success throughout the different areas of your life.

How Childhood Adversity Impacts the Body

Research has clearly shown that adverse experiences, unresolved emotions, and events from childhood don't just make a mark on our memories; they have a lasting impact on the body. In his book *The Biology of Belief,* author Bruce Lipton, Ph.D., explains why early childhood has such a significant impact on our emotional, mental, and physical well-being throughout our adult years:

> The fundamental behaviors, beliefs, and attitudes we observe in our parents become "hard-wired" as synaptic pathways in our subconscious minds. Once programmed into the subconscious mind, they control our biology for the rest of our lives . . . unless we can figure out a way to reprogram them. Anyone who doubts the sophistication of this downloading should think about the first time your child blurted out a curse word picked up from you. I'm sure you noted its sophistication, correct pronunciation, its nuanced style, and context carrying your signature.
>
> Given the precision of this behavior-recording system, imagine the consequences of hearing your parents say you are a "stupid child," you "do not deserve things," will "never amount to anything," "never should have been born," or are a "sickly, weak" person. When unthinking or uncaring parents pass on those messages to their young children, they are no doubt oblivious to the fact that such comments are downloaded into the subconscious memory as absolute "facts" just as surely as bits and bytes are downloaded to the hard drive of your desktop computer. During early development, the child's consciousness has not evolved enough to critically assess that those parental pronouncements were only verbal barbs and not necessarily true characterizations of "self." Once programmed into the subconscious mind, however, these verbal abuses become defined as "truths" that unconsciously shape the behavior and potential of the child through life.

The Adverse Childhood Experiences (ACE Study), a research project funded by Kaiser Permanente and the Centers for Disease Control, confirms the lasting impact of early childhood. The ACE Study, which followed more than 17,000 participants, found that unresolved childhood trauma has profound effects on the body well into adulthood. Compared with someone with an ACE score of 0, a person with a high ACE score is nearly three times more likely to smoke and a whopping 30 times more likely to attempt suicide. The study also confirmed direct correlations between childhood trauma and cancer, heart disease, diabetes, stroke, high blood pressure, bone fracture, depression, and drug use. Many of the study participants were over 60 years of age, which indicates that childhood trauma and adverse experiences continue to impact the body decades after they take place.

The ACE Study findings are confirmed by Renee D. Goodwin and Murray B. Stein's 2004 study called "Association Between Childhood Trauma and Physical Disorders Among Adults in the United States." It states:

> Childhood physical abuse, sexual abuse and neglect were associated with a statistically significantly increased risk of a wide range of physical illnesses during adulthood. After adjusting for demographic characteristics, lifetime anxiety and depressive disorders, alcohol and substance dependence, and all types of trauma: results showed that childhood physical abuse was associated with increased risk of lung disease, peptic ulcer and arthritic disorders, childhood sexual abuse was associated with increased risk of cardiac disease and childhood neglect was associated with increased risk of diabetes and autoimmune disorders.

As we'll see in the following pages, these connections between childhood adversity and disease also apply to chronic pain.

Big T and Little t

The events and circumstances that can contribute to chronic pain in adulthood span a wide range. As my friend and EFT expert Carol Look says, "There's trauma with a little *t,* and trauma with a big *T.*"

Big-T trauma refers to major events—an accident, sexual abuse, or the loss of a parent or sibling. Little-t trauma is often less noticeable, like being bullied at school or living with an emotionally unavailable parent. All of these occurrences can leave emotional scars that impact the body in adulthood. Particularly when they stem from childhood, repressed emotions and unresolved experiences put the body on chronic high alert. As we've seen, over time that "stressed state" gradually wears your body down, interfering with the body's ability to heal itself and putting you at greater risk for chronic pain. As Rick Hanson, Ph.D., author of *Hardwiring Happiness,* explains, "Alarming or painful life experiences, especially traumatic ones, naturally make a person more fearful. If you grew up in a dangerous neighborhood, had angry or unpredictable parents, or were bullied in school, it's normal to still be watchful even if you now live in a safe place with nice people."

As we explore childhood memories and experiences, it's important for you to be aware of what seems too big to handle on your own. While EFT is a safe and effective way to process and release trauma, if you find yourself feeling unsafe or overwhelmed while trying to work through your past, stop and seek the support of a psychologist or therapist who has been trained in using EFT to overcome trauma. You can find a list of professionals who use EFT in their practices at thetappingsolution.com/eft-practitioners. (This list includes both coaches and clinical practitioners, so make sure to find someone who has experience and training in dealing with trauma specifically.)

Similarly, if you have a friend or family member who wants to use EFT to overcome past trauma that seems like too much to process on their own, take the same precaution and seek out a trained professional first.

Even Happy Childhoods Aren't Perfect

The most noticeable thing about Sylvia, as compared with the majority of my clients, was her age. At 28 years old, she'd had chronic pain in her arms for almost ten years, and in her feet for more than three years. Hoping for relief, she'd submitted an application to work with me.

When I first asked Sylvia about her childhood, she shrugged and said she'd had a pretty normal one. Most of her time growing up had been dedicated to sports, especially basketball, she explained. Her pain had begun in college, during the endless hours she'd spent studying alone in the library. She'd get settled in the library early in the morning and stay until dinner, often skipping lunch to get more done. "Why did you push yourself so hard?" I asked her. "I guess I was trying to be perfect," she answered.

College was the first time Sylvia hadn't played basketball, she explained, and she had channeled all her effort into getting top grades. "I feel like I always have to be perfect at something," she added. "Before college, I always had to be perfect at basketball, but college was the first time I didn't play basketball, so I focused all my time and energy on my grades."

"Whom are you trying to be perfect for?" I asked her.

"My dad," she answered. "He's never been happy enough with me."

When I asked her why she thought that, tears rolled down her cheeks as her voice began to quake. "My dad was also the coach of my basketball team," she said with a quick nervous laugh.

One of her first memories with her dad was from when she was 11 years old, playing basketball. It wasn't a particularly important game, but the score was tied, and her dad was tense. During a time-out in the final minutes of the game, Sylvia got into a huddle with her dad and teammates. With everyone looking on, her dad pointed his finger directly at her and said that it was up to her to win the game.

"How did that make you feel?" I asked her.

"Angry," she said as she tapped through the points.

"Also sad that I have a dad who was more focused on winning the game than anything else," she added.

Instead of expressing how she felt at that moment, though, Sylvia had kept quiet and focused on making the winning baskets her dad wanted. She had succeeded, but shortly after the game ended, Sylvia had begun to hyperventilate and had to be rushed to the hospital. That was the start of a years-long pattern, she said. Throughout high school, she would hyperventilate after games fairly often, even when she'd played really well.

ASK YOURSELF: Did you experience any physical symptoms as a kid? If so, your body may have been trying to get your attention! Make note of any childhood symptoms you experienced in your journal, including what activities you were doing, whom you were with, and so on, when the symptoms appeared. Then be sure to tap through those memories and release any remaining emotional charge.

I began guiding Sylvia through several rounds of tapping on her anger at her dad, and then asked her to visualize that moment in the team huddle, but this time to say and do what she'd wanted to. "Have some fun with it," I told her. "Say anything and everything you wanted to say that day."

Tapping while imagining talking to her dad at that moment, she began, "It's just a stupid game, Dad. It's not that big of a deal. Stop pressuring me."

I then asked her to visualize herself grabbing his clipboard. "Start smacking him around with it in front of everyone at the game," I suggested. She laughed and continued to speak to him, voicing her anger and sadness at all the pressure he'd put on her to perform over the years. Although at no point did we tap specifically on her physical pain, by the end of our session, Sylvia's foot and arm pain had gone from an 8 out of 10 down to a 4 out of 10.

Sylvia's story is a great example of how seemingly small events in childhood can get lodged in the body and contribute to physical pain in adulthood. Because of her dad's dissatisfaction with her basketball game at 11 years old, Sylvia had created a belief that she was not good enough and always needed to try harder and do more. Although her dad's behavior on the court wasn't good, she'd experienced no major traumas and otherwise had enjoyed a fairly good childhood. "My dad's not a bad guy," she later shared. "He also has a really good, caring side." What had stayed in her body, however, was the anger and sadness she'd never expressed to him on the basketball court.

Most of us experienced similar kinds of pressure or stress at some point in childhood. To this day, I still vividly remember the time I locked myself in the car at school at seven years old. We had recently moved to the United States from Argentina, and while I had a supportive and loving family and a great childhood in many other ways, during that period of time, I was miserable at school. I felt like an outcast and dreaded going every day. Locking myself in the car was my way of expressing the anger I felt for having to spend so much time in a place where I felt isolated.

Fortunately, several months later, we moved to a different area, where I attended a school that I loved. I quickly made new friends there and had a great time, but those first months in America were really challenging. At seven years old, experiences like that feel traumatic. The good news is, I've been tapping for all these years, ridding my body of that negative emotional energy.

Releasing the Past: Personal Peace Procedure

Now it's time to begin looking at events in your childhood that may be connected to your chronic pain in some way. One great exercise for this kind of exploration is the Personal Peace Procedure, which was developed by Gary Craig.

This exercise involves making a list of every bothersome specific event in your life and systematically tapping on them. While this exercise can be used for all periods of your life, for now we will focus only on your childhood. As you discover, neutralize, and eliminate the emotional baggage from specific childhood events, you will, of course, have less and less internal conflict for your body to deal with.

Less internal conflict translates into a higher level of personal peace and less emotional and physical suffering, all of which supports pain relief.

The steps are as follows:

1. In your journal, make a list of all the bothersome events from childhood. Don't be surprised if you find yourself with a fairly long list! That's normal. It's often helpful to chunk time into segments to help jog your memory:

   - Birth, 0–5 years old, 5–10 years old, 10–15, and 15–18.

   - Relationships with siblings or anyone else who lived in the house with you.

   - Your school experience: kindergarten–first grade, elementary school, junior high school, high school, college.

   - Other traumas, illnesses, accidents, hospitalizations.

   - The nature of relationships: with your mother, your father, friends, other significant relationships.

   - What did you learn or tell yourself from these events and relationships about yourself, about others, or about the world? Remember, you can tap and clear the negative beliefs you took on as a result of these events.

2. While making your list, you may find that some events don't seem to cause you any current discomfort. That's okay. List them anyway. The fact that you remember them suggests a need for resolution.

3. Give them all a 0–10 rating (10 is the highest level of emotional intensity).

4. Starting with the 10s, tap through each of them. Be sure to notice any specific aspects that may come up and tap on those, as well. You might start by working on one issue from an event, such as anger, and then find that another "aspect" comes up, such as sadness.

5. As you tap, new memories or concerns might come up; give them a number and add them to the list.

By developing a practice of tapping on a daily basis, working on two to three events on your list, you can easily address dozens, even hundreds, of specific events in a few months. Take note in a journal of any changes you've noticed, such as how your body feels, where you feel pain and how intensely, how often you get upset or triggered, and the shifts and changes in your relationships. Revisit some of those specific events and notice how those previously intense incidents have faded into nothingness.

As we'll see next, sometimes it's the words people say to us as children that contribute most to chronic pain.

When Hurtful Words Stick with Us

For Bobbie, the pain had begun 25 years earlier, soon after her dad died. "There was so much rage I wanted to express for what he put us through growing up, and I didn't get the chance. And I didn't get the chance to hear my father say that he was proud of me, and that was the one thing I wanted to hear in my life more than anything. I tried my hardest, and I never got that."

It was the second day of a live pain-relief event, and we'd just begun the hard work of digging into the past. Bobbie had volunteered to come onstage. Almost as soon as she began speaking, tears started to stream down her cheeks. "I was told at the age of five by my dad," she began, "that he wished I'd never been born . . . and on my birthday . . . He spent the rest of his life making sure I understood how much I didn't matter and how little I was worth. I heard every day of my life that I was a fat, useless, lazy slob that no one could ever love."

"Why did he do that?" I asked her.

"Because he didn't know better. He never had it himself, so he didn't know how to give it . . . and all I wanted was his love. I came home with a straight-A report card, and my father asked me how many of my teachers I'd had to sleep with to get those grades."

The audience gasped in horror.

"I was in junior high, and I'd gotten those grades because I wanted my father to be proud of me," she continued. "That was the first time I realized that I wanted him to be proud of me," she added, sobbing quietly.

"When he died, I lost that chance. And I had a little boy, he was just six months old, and the pain started limiting me from being able to play with him, to the point where when he was two years old, and my husband asked me what I wanted for my birthday, I said, 'If you really want to get me what I want for my birthday, go grab one of your shotguns and shoot me.' And I meant it with every fiber of my being. I just didn't want be here anymore. My son was sitting next to me on the couch. I wanted to be gone because if my own father couldn't love me, what hope was there?"

Bobbie kept tapping, sobbing as the memories flooded back. "I'm just so angry with him . . . and I've stuffed it down my whole life."

To begin neutralizing the memories of her dad, I slowly began walking Bobbie through her memory.

"What did he look like?" I asked.

"Average height, average build, you know, just a hardworking man," she replied, still tapping.

"What was his job?" I asked.

"He was a head machinist at a paper converting [factory] in Green Bay," she replied.

"What's your youngest memory of him?" I asked.

She then began telling the story of when her dad told her he wished she'd never been born. "I was five; it was on my birthday. He said it in front of my friends, and I got up and ran into the bathroom. I crawled into the tub and just started rocking back and forth," she said.

"Where do you see that memory now? Is it a picture? Do you feel it in your body?" I asked.

"It's right here," she replied, pointing to her stomach. "It's just tight. There's this locked door that's got to hold it down, because if I open it up, what do I feel?" she said.

"So it's behind a locked door?" I asked.

"A very solid door . . . Six or seven inches [thick], at least," she answered.

"Is it wood? Metal? How do you open and close it?" I asked, prompting her to complete the picture in her mind. "It's metal," she said. "There's no handle."

Once we finished visualizing the door blocking her from her emotions, I returned to the birthday. "How many people were at your birthday party?" I asked.

"Three or four, and my mom. She came and got me in the bathroom, and she pulled the curtain back, and said, 'Honey, it's okay. It's okay. He didn't mean it. He was drinking again. Just come out. We'll have some cake—that'll make it all better,'" she explained.

We'd covered several segments of her fifth birthday party, but not in sequential order. To release more of the emotional charge from that event, I wanted to give her a chance to relive her memory from start to finish. "Tell me about the start of the birthday party," I said.

"It was just at the kitchen table," she replied. "That was the last birthday party I ever had." I asked her to picture where she was sitting at the table. "I'm sitting at the kitchen table with my friends," she began, "with my back to the hallway that leads out to the garage."

I asked her to pause the story. "See yourself there. How did that little girl feel in that moment?" I asked.

"I was really happy," she sobbed. "We were laughing and joking. And then the door shut, and my dad came in. And I could smell the beer before he got to me," she said.

"What happens when you smell the beer? How do you feel?" I asked.

"I start getting scared, because Dad embarrassed us a lot," she said.

"Pause there. Do you feel that happiness fade away?" I asked.

"It was gone immediately," she said. "At five, I was thinking, *Where's my escape route and what can I do to stop this from happening?* Something was going to happen; I just knew it."

"Feel that fear in your body. Where do you feel that fear, just of smelling the beer? Don't go any further," I said.

"In my chest, and in my stomach . . . and my knee is hurting right now," she added.

"How strong is that fear in your chest and stomach?" I asked.

"A seven," she said.

"And what's the fear about? What going to happen next?" I asked.

"What he's going to do, what he's going to say . . . because dad never hit us. He wasn't allowed to hit us. That was one rule my mom had—you're not allowed to touch those kids," she said, remembering what her mom used to tell him.

We did some tapping on Bobbie's fear of what her dad was going to say. "Even though I have all this fear in my body . . . of what Dad is going to say . . . I choose to relax and feel safe now," we began. "All this fear," we continued as we tapped through the points. "What's he going to say? . . . I need to hide . . . this isn't safe." To begin defusing her fear, I ended our tapping with "I am safe now . . . the five-year-old in me is safe . . . that part of me is safe . . . right now."

Often, when we return to challenging memories from childhood, we become the vulnerable little child we were then, which is an important part of the healing process. However, when we're in that place, it's also important to retrain the brain to step back and remember that we're no longer facing that same threat. We're adults now, capable of defending and protecting ourselves in ways we couldn't as children.

When we were done tapping, to test our results with the fear she felt upon smelling the beer, I asked Bobbie to rewind to the beginning of the party again, and tell me one more time about the good feelings at the beginning of the party. "We were joking around and having fun," she began, able to smile as she spoke this time. "And my brother was there," she added. "I hadn't remembered him being there until just now," she said, pleasantly surprised.

"So you're having fun," I said, "and you smell beer on your dad's breath. How does that feel in your body?" I asked.

"I still feel the tightness," she replied. "It's about a three or four." Her fear had gone from a 7 down to a 3 or 4, so I asked her to go further.

"He walks up behind me and puts his hands on my shoulders, and . . . " She stopped as the tears began to flow again.

"Pause there," I said once again.

When we're tapping through deeply rooted childhood experiences, it's important to take it slowly. To release the full emotional charge from events like this, stop and tap on each point in the story that carries a strong emotional charge. Keep tapping until you clear, or significantly lower, the intensity of each emotionally charged moment in the memory before moving forward. (This is why working with a practitioner can be helpful, to guide you through every step of an event like this.)

"He's got his hands on your shoulders. How does that make you feel?" I continued.

"I know what's coming next, so it hurts," she said, beginning to sob.

I started another round of tapping. "Even though I know what's coming next, and it hurts so much . . . I heard it then . . . and I've been hearing it every day since then . . . I know exactly what's next . . . when I feel those hands on my shoulders . . . but I choose to relax . . . and feel safe now." We did several rounds of tapping on the anxiety she felt when her dad's hands were on her shoulders. "Here we go . . . life-changing event . . . about to happen . . . I feel it coming . . . and I'm scared . . . because it's going to go . . . to the root of my being . . . it's going to stab me through the heart . . . this pain that's coming up."

When we were done with that round of tapping, I restarted the story of her birthday party. When I got to the part about smelling beer on her dad's breath,

I asked her how she felt. "I don't feel anything now. There's no tightening or anything when I smell it." When I got to the part where her dad put his hands on her shoulders, I asked her how anxious she felt. "Just a little bit, like a two," she replied.

Since the emotional charge of both of those moments had gone away or lowered significantly, I asked her what was next. "His hands are on my shoulders, and I look up into his face because there was a squeeze, like he wanted me to look up. So I'm looking up into my father's face, and we're only that far apart," she said, her hands indicating a space of a couple of feet between their faces.

• •

When we're tapping through deeply rooted childhood experiences, it's important to take it slowly. To release the full emotional charge from events like this, stop and tap on each point in the story that carries a strong emotional charge. Keep tapping until you clear, or significantly lower, the intensity of each emotionally charged moment in the memory before moving forward.

• •

Her tears began to flow again, so I began another round of tapping. "Even though I know what's about to happen, I choose to relax and feel safe now . . . even though I know what I'm about to hear . . . it's going to devastate me . . . and I wish for this thing to not happen . . . I wish I'd run away . . . I wish I'd thrown cake in his face." We both laughed and continued tapping. "Anything for this not to happen . . . I choose to relax and feel safe now."

I asked her how she felt when she looked up at her dad now. "I don't feel anything when I look up now. No fear or anything," she said.

"Okay, what happened next?" I asked.

"I looked up, and I can feel this hope that he'd wish me a happy birthday, because my dad never even knew when our birthdays were. He didn't believe in them . . . And, uh, he took his cigar out of his mouth, so I can smell that," she continued. "And he just looked me in the eyes, straight in the eyes, not even looking away, and said, 'I wish you had never been born.'"

I asked her how she felt when she hears that now. "The door slammed shut," she said.

"Oh, the door was open before?" I asked.

"Yeah, it was open," she said, about to continue telling more of the story.

"Let's back it up," I said. We began tapping. "This door's about to slam shut, because I'm about to hear these words . . . but I choose to relax and feel safe . . . even though he's about to say some terrible things, I choose to relax . . . and feel safe, and know that nothing that he's about to say . . . is true . . . everything he's about to say . . . is a lie . . . but it's going to hurt . . . because I'm five."

When we were back at the eyebrow point, I asked her to say each word slowly, one at a time, and tap on one point with each word. She began, "God . . . I . . . wish . . . you . . . had . . . never . . . been . . . born." I asked her how she felt when she said that.

"Mad," she said. "I've always been hurt, but now I'm mad." This kind of shift is a really good sign, as we've seen. I asked her what she wanted to say to him now.

"Can you edit this?" she asked, laughing with the audience. I smiled and nodded. "How," she began, "could anyone look into the eyes of an innocent five-year-old child and tell them they wish they'd never been born? . . . I loved you with all of my heart . . . What a horrible seed to plant in a child."

She then called him all the names everyone in the room wanted to call him by that point. "Why do I still love you? You don't deserve it," she continued. "I didn't get yours, you don't deserve mine," she cried. "I was the one who made everything okay in the house and protected everyone."

Next I asked her to visualize where the cake was. "Can you think of some things you'd like to do with that cake?" I asked. She laughed.

"I can think of the things I can do with my elbow. I wanted to hurt him where it hurt most. I wanted to see him drop to his knees, at my level."

I told her to imagine herself as an ironclad five-year-old. "No one can hurt you," I told her. "Do what you want to do."

Her left elbow jutted backward. Bobbie was the second or third person to imagine punching a dad where it hurts most, so I joked, "This is punching- guys-in-the-balls weekend . . . It's a new therapy." We all laughed.

"Then I throw the cake at him," Bobbie continued, throwing her elbow backward again, and then motioning her arms as if she was tossing the cake overhead to land on her father, who, in her visualization, was now in a pile on the floor behind her.

"Now he sulks away," I said, prompting her to continue.

"Now he's mad," she said.

"It's okay. You're made of steel. He can't touch you," I reminded her.

She nodded. "He storms off," she said. I asked her to take me back to the door she'd seen earlier. "Now it's transparent," she said, "and the little girl in there is smiling . . . she's smiling . . . wow," Bobbie said, smiling herself.

I asked her what it would take to get that little girl out of there. "Finally saying he was wrong and feeling it everywhere . . . because I've said he was wrong and I've worked on it before, but not like this," she said. I asked her what it would take to feel that. "I don't know," she replied.

Letting my intuition lead the way, I asked for an extra microphone onstage, and asked Bobbie to stand up and move toward front and center onstage. She seemed hesitant, but she did it anyway. I handed the microphone to Thomas, who was sitting in the front row.

"He was wrong," he began, and passed the microphone to his neighbor in the audience. For the next 15 minutes, the microphone passed from one audience member to the next as each one told Bobbie that her dad had been wrong. She cried as she listened, tapping through the points the entire time. When the last person was done, I came back onstage and asked Bobbie how the little girl was doing. "She's not in there anymore," she said.

After lunch, Bobbie came back onstage to share her results. "I was telling my roommate Nikki that I don't have knee pain, and it's been twenty-five years of pain," she said in amazement. She thanked the audience for the love they'd shared with her. I asked her what no knee pain meant to her and her future. "I can walk forward into my future now," she said as the audience clapped and howled.

I asked her to retell the story of her fifth birthday party. With no tears, and at times, even a smile on her face, she retold the story in a matter-of-fact way. "Now I get that it was never about me," she added. "He was a lost man, and he had to hurt someone as much as he hurt. And then I went back into my party and enjoyed myself," she laughed. "And the steel door, after it became transparent, opened and then disappeared. And it's gone completely."

The following morning, Bobbie came back up onstage to share her experience of going to New York City the night before. "I went up and down stairs in Grand Central Station that I never would have attempted before this, because I would have thought, first of all, I'm too fat to walk up those stairs, and second of all, my knees will hurt too badly by the time I'm done," she began. "And none of that went through my head. I went up those stairs like nothing," she said as the audience clapped.

When she'd gotten back to her room later that night, she added, she got into her normal sleeping position in bed and heard herself groaning, as if she was in pain. "But there was no pain," she said. "And the same thing happened this morning when getting out of bed. I made that noise, but then said to myself, *What are you making that noise for? It doesn't hurt.*" She laughed, as the audience once again broke out in applause.

Watch Bobbie's Session, Live! To watch the video of Bobbie's session live, visit: thetappingsolution.com/painbookresources.

Even with her brain still programmed to expect pain last thing at night and first thing in the morning, Bobbie felt no pain. It was such a clear demonstration of how the pain isn't just about the pain. It's about the expectation of pain and the pattern and emotional charge behind the pain. And when you clear those patterns, release that emotional charge, the pain can go away even when your brain still expects the pain to appear.

A Recap of Bobbie's Session

Here are the steps we used to process and clear the emotional charge of this memory from Bobbie's childhood:

1. First, I had her tell her story while tapping. This is always the best place to start, because it gives you a chance to unearth any memories, thoughts, and feelings that may have been buried in your subconscious mind. Just say whatever comes to mind, without editing yourself or trying to adhere to any method or technique. At this stage of the process, you want to begin to let it all out.

2. As her emotional intensity began to build, I began to lead Bobbie through the Movie Technique. I had her visualize each part of the story,

---

beginning with what her dad looked like. This technique brings all your senses into the experience, incorporating visual memories as well as memories of sound, smell, and touch. By involving as many different sensory components as possible, you're bringing your memory back to life more vividly. That makes your tapping more powerful, so you can then clear the emotional charge more fully and in less time.

3. As she began to connect with her emotions around the memory—the "movie" we were running—I asked her where in her body she felt this memory. For Bobbie, the "movie" was behind a thick, solid metal door. For another person, it could be tightness in the stomach, stabbing pain in a certain body part, numbness, or something else. Whatever it is, try to identify where in your body you feel this memory and associate that feeling with a visual, if you can.

4. As we progressed through the "movie," we paused to tap on each emotionally charged moment in the story. Throughout her "movie," I also had her identify where in her body she felt each challenging emotion. We made sure to clear the emotional charge of each difficult point before moving on in the "movie."

5. When we got to the emotional climax of the story—the point at which her dad said the words, "God, I wish you had never been born"—I had her slow down and say one word at a time, tapping on only one point for each word. She did this for a few rounds to begin clearing the emotional charge of these words that had haunted her for most of her life.

6. Once we'd tapped through and cleared the most painful parts of her story, I added humor and fun into the process by having her visualize throwing cake at her dad. Whenever it feels right, try to make the process enjoyable. This is so important! Incorporating humor and levity can be incredibly healing, allowing you to take your power back in ways that feel good.

7. Finally, to pry open the thick, solid metal door that her emotions had been locked behind, I used the power of group energy, passing the microphone around the audience to have them tell her what she needed to hear—that her dad was wrong. While this exact exercise isn't

> possible when you're tapping on your own, you can access a similar healing energy with groups of supportive friends, whether in person or online through social media. If you do choose to try this, be absolutely certain first that the people you pick are willing to support you and your process without judgment or criticism. This is a time for complete acceptance and 100 percent support.
>
> Remember: Throughout the process, every time we cleared an emotionally charged "peak" moment, we began the story again to test our results. This is crucial! You need to revisit the earlier parts of the story and check in to see if the emotional charge is still there. If earlier parts of your story—your "movie"—still feel upsetting in any way, keep tapping on that moment until you can retell that part of the story without the emotional charge.

Struggling with How to Tap on Your Own? If you feel unsure about how to tap on your own, go back and watch my "How to Tap for Pain Relief" video at: thetappingsolution.com/painbookresources.

Releasing Traumatic Childhood Memories

For the first time during the entire weekend of my pain-relief event, several men (who are sometimes in short supply at transformational events!) raised their hands to share their stories. One of them was Mark. "Yesterday when we were working through what we thought was the initial pain event, I kept going back to something that happened eight years ago," he began, fighting back tears. I asked him to start tapping.

"Somebody said to me yesterday that they wanted to see a man get up there and cry, and I'm a people pleaser," he joked.

"Okay, hold on," I said. "We're going with men today. Let's get some men up here . . . We need a few good men leading the way," I added, remarking on how many more women than men were in the audience.

Will I Ever Get All My Tapping Done?

I know I've been showing you how to peel back the layers, and by this time you may be wondering how you're ever going to get to the bottom of it all. Know that you don't have to do it all in one sitting. You may find that you work on one aspect of an event, you get the charge down to a 2 or lower, and then you take a break. The next time you look at that event, you notice that there is a different aspect to it that you focus on and you tap it down again to a 2 or lower. With patience and persistence, you'll eventually get all the aspects around that event down to 0.

Once he was settled onstage, I asked Mark to start tapping while continuing his story of what had happened eight years before. It had been a difficult time, he shared, and he'd ruptured a disc while working in the garden. Ever since, he'd had pain in his lower back and in his shoulders. "Things were going on at that time that were challenging from a work perspective, from a financial perspective, that kind of thing," he explained, "but something kept popping into my head from when I was twelve or thirteen years old, and it's something I've been working on, but it's not something I'd attributed the pain to . . . and when I started tapping on that, it dredged up a bunch of events that are all connected to one particular day, and shortly after that day is when I hurt my lower back . . . and I'd never before connected all of those together."

Mark paused, clearly struggling to hold back his emotions. "And it has to do with . . . the fact that I was physically abused by my father growing up and sexually abused by an older boy." His voice quaked as his eyes filled with tears. "That's not something that men talk a lot about, because, you know, we're men . . . and I'd been working on those issues with other professionals, but I'd never connected it to the pain until I went back to this one day," he said.

"The abuse from my father was bad," he continued. "You didn't come to him for anything; you didn't show problems or ask for any help. I heard the phrase 'I'll give you something to cry about' a lot, and he sure gave us something to cry about in a very alarming way. This wasn't just the strap; it was weird things, his punishments, so he sure gave us things to cry about . . . So you never cracked, you never showed pressure, and you were always scared that you'd do something wrong." He took a deep breath.

"And then the day that I identified," he shared as tears began to flow. "And the older boy was with me, and my older brother walked in. The first words out of his mouth weren't, *What's going on here?* The first words out of his mouth were, *Don't worry, Mark, I won't tell Dad* . . . twelve years old, and that was when the blinders came off . . . and when I hit this point, huge amounts of rage . . . shame . . . fear . . . and my back started tightening up," he shared.

"And I've been experimenting with that, and as I focus on that day, my lower left back starts tightening up, and the rage, shame, and fear come . . . I'm stuck on this. And I have two boys, ages ten and seven, and every time I look at them, I see me at that age, and I know what was going on . . . and I kept it all in a box until my boys showed up, and I began to see my little boy, and what might happen to him . . . and I think that's where the pain all started."

I asked Mark which emotion stood out most, the rage, shame, or fear. "It's one word—rage/shame/fear. It's electric. It goes all the way through my body. There's the pain spot that's there all the time. But when I connected all of these events with the pain yesterday, when it hit, it's like I'm holding on to two electrical wires. It's just . . . everywhere."

I then gently guided Mark back to that day when his older brother had walked in as the other older boy was molesting him. "That day pulls it all together. That's the day it stopped," he said. "I don't know when it started."

I asked him if there was a picture of that day, what the room looked like, what his brother was wearing. He closed his eyes tightly, fighting back more tears. Nodding in response to my question, he said quietly, "I remember everything."

Seeing the pain on Mark's face, I began a tapping round. "Even though I have all this rage, shame, and fear in my body . . . about that day . . . my brother walked in . . . on that terrible situation," I began. When we got to "I deeply and completely love and accept myself," Mark went silent.

During the next round, I offered "I accept part of me" as a substitute phrase. We continued tapping on all the rage, shame, and fear coursing through his body. "That terrible day . . . when my brother walked in . . . and that terrible situation . . . I'm so ashamed . . . I'm so angry . . . all this rage . . . how could this happen? . . . I see my boys now . . . and I see myself at that age . . . so young . . . so vulnerable . . . it was so wrong . . . all this anger . . . all this shame . . . all this fear . . . in my body . . . it's time to let it go."

When we were done, I brought him back to that day. I asked him to begin tapping on the eyebrow point again. "What did you feel when your brother opened that door?" I asked.

"I'm afraid," he began. "Afraid I'm in trouble, afraid my father's going to find out."

I asked him what would happen if his father found out.

"I don't know," he said. "Somebody would be beat." He began to cry.

The fear Mark had felt at that moment was still very real, so I led him through several rounds focused specifically on the moment when his brother opened the door. We tapped on his fear and on the shame he felt about what his brother saw. I ended with "But it's safe to accept myself, even with all those terrible days . . . even with what happened . . . and how I was abused."

When we were done, Mark's electricity was a 2 or 3 out of 10, down from an 8 out of 10. He pictured his brother opening the door and didn't feel any fear. His memory of that day included several other emotionally charged moments, so I asked him to keep tapping through the points while visualizing everything he could recall from that day. He didn't need to say anything out loud, just to see it in his mind, and to try to stay aware of the tightness, pain, and electricity in his body as he did so.

It's important to feel supported when we're working through trauma, so as he imagined that day, I continued to guide him through it. "See what happened," I began. "Feel what you felt." With his eyes closed, he continued tapping, breathing heavily as tears streamed down his face.

At several moments, he was visibly overwhelmed by emotion as he played the movie through in his mind. "Feel how safe it is," I offered, "to feel these feelings." I continued talking throughout. Once he seemed to have worked through the most intense parts of his memory, I began to bring him back to the present moment. "You are loved," I offered. "Even though all these terrible things happened, you are loved. See that younger version of you, see any remaining pain or shame, rage, and fear that he felt, and you can just tell him, 'You are loved.' Go ahead and see yourself telling him that. Everything's going to be okay."

After several minutes of tapping, Mark's face began to relax. I asked him to visualize all the places in his body where he'd stored his rage, shame, and fear, and to begin seeing them being filled with love, love for himself, acceptance of himself. I asked him to feel how his body responds to that love, hope, and joy, and how all the inflammation goes down and all the muscles relax, loosen, and breathe for the first time.

After tapping through that memory, I asked him to stop tapping and take a deep breath, breathe into any remaining tightness and tension, and let it go while feeling love for himself in his heart.

"Just know that this is you," I said. "This is you at your strongest, you at your bravest. This is what it means to be a man. Love in your heart. Acceptance of yourself. Courage to move forward and heal. This is what it means to be a man. Not whatever your dad taught you. Not that old outdated model of what it means to be a man. Feel that strength, that courage, that peace."

After a couple of minutes talking him through this visualization, I asked Mark to open his eyes when he felt ready. When he did, the electricity in his body was gone, and his back pain had gone down to a 1 out of 10. He began moving around in the chair, bending forward and to each side. "There seems to be flexibility that wasn't there before," he shared. The audience clapped and howled with excitement.

"As I said, I've been stuck, and I don't know how to get beyond the navel-gazing about what happened in that room," he shared, "and what you just took me through was helpful because . . . I deal with my sons from a place of love, kindness, and respect for them, not fear and pain. I've never dealt with myself that way," he added, beginning to get choked up.

"This time I'm just getting emotional, not freaked out," he said, as the audience laughed along with him. "I've never dealt with my [inner] eight-year-old boy the way I deal with my eight-year-old son," he continued, "and I think that will help going forward." The audience broke out in applause once again.

Traumatic memories like Mark's often replay in our minds over and over again, even after decades have passed. Since, by definition, the experience of revisiting trauma, mentally and/or emotionally, doesn't feel safe, I urge you to seek out the support of a professional before delving into traumatic memories like these. A professional can guide you, step by step, through the process, as I did for Mark. That person can also make sure that you have cleared the emotional charge fully and then end with a positive visualization, which is so important for grounding yourself back in the present.

For Mark I felt it was important that he create a new definition of himself as the new model of a "real man," one who has the courage to feel his emotions and accept and love himself. Because he had cleared the emotional charge of his memories by recalling them while tapping through the points, these positive visualizations allowed Mark to ground himself in the man he is now, rather than getting lost in painful parts of his past.

The Pain-Empathy Connection

When pain expert Sean Mackey, associate professor and chief of the Pain Management Division of Stanford University Medical Center, arrived at his five-year-old son's school and saw his son fall hard and hit his head while running very fast toward him, Mackey felt a physical jolt in his body. As his son's head hit the floor, Mackey heard a loud thud that caused him and all the parents nearby to gasp in horror. When Mackey ran to his son's side and asked him if he was okay, his son said he was fine, and then high-fived his dad.

Although a goose egg immediately began growing on his head, his son didn't appear to be feeling much pain. Mackey realized at that moment that he might have experienced as much or more pain watching his son fall than his son had felt. As a result of that experience, Mackey's team at Stanford did a study about the relationship between empathy and pain.

In the study, participants' brain activity was continuously monitored via fMRI. At one point participants were exposed to thermal pain on one arm that was a 7 out of 10 in intensity. At a different time, participants were hooked up to fMRI while they watched especially graphic videos of people being injured, mostly in professional sports games, so imagine watching an athlete's limb being contorted as you hear a loud snapping noise. These were brutally graphic injuries that happened suddenly, with no warning.

During both experiences—while participants were being exposed to physical thermal pain and while they were watching the videos of people being injured—similar parts of the brain, regions involved in emotional as well as cognitive processing, were activated. The findings suggest that by empathizing with another person's pain, we are able to feel it to some degree.

Gaining Freedom from the Past

When we're willing to do this work and use tapping to clear the emotional pain of childhood memories that haven't faded with time, pain relief is often the first step in a much larger process. As we'll see later in this book, without this heavy emotional baggage from childhood weighing on us, our lives often change in incredible ways.

Audio Bonus: My sister, Jessica, who made the original *Tapping Solution* film with me and is now the *New York Times* best-selling author of *The Tapping Solution for Weight Loss and Body Confidence,* has been sharing a "Personal Peace" meditation during our annual Tapping World Summits for several years. It's gotten rave reviews and I'd like to share it with you here: thetappingsolution.com/painbookresources.

CHAPTER 8

CLEARING RESISTANCE TO CHANGE: WHEN WE BECOME OUR PAIN

Let's move on to something completely different now. We've looked at our pasts, our traumas, and our experiences that may have influenced our pain and that keep our pain stuck. But now let's look at the present. What would be different if your pain went away? What would change for the better, and what would change for the worse? In this chapter, we'll explore the downsides to pain relief and the upsides to pain.

Already, I can hear your mental wheels turning . . . an upside to pain? Downside to pain relief? Huh? Even the subtitle of this chapter—"When We Become Our Pain"—may have you scratching your head. The only thing you want is pain relief. That's the whole reason you're reading this book!

The topic we're discussing in this chapter isn't obvious or straightforward. It's controlled by the unconscious mind, so we're rarely aware it's happening.

The Subversive Power of the Unconscious Mind

When the pain hits, you just want it to go away. You want to feel good. You want to live a life where pain isn't the first thing you think about in the morning and the last thing you think about at night. That's your conscious mind, screaming for pain relief.

Your unconscious mind is a lot trickier. As we've seen, its job is to protect you, and in carrying out that role, it can subvert and sabotage the desires of your conscious mind. This powerful process happens inside all of us.

I experienced this struggle in regard to my financial success. A few years out of college, I hit my stride with a growing web development and marketing consulting business. At the time, I was earning triple what many of my friends were making. To celebrate that success, I put together a weeklong vacation in two stunning villas in Mexico with 12 of my closest friends. We had an incredible time, and to this day, I still enjoy thinking back on all the great memories from that trip.

The following year, I tried to schedule a similar trip, but the same villas weren't available. As a result, each person would have to pay more to go this time around. Several friends bowed out, saying they couldn't afford the trip. I called several others, hoping to convince them to come. One friend responded by saying, "We don't all make as much money as you do. We can't just do whatever we want." It was a tough conversation, and I hung up feeling bad about making more money than my friends did. Was my financial success making people mad at me? Jealous? Was I losing friends because of it?

Though I was unaware that my unconscious mind had taken over as a result of that conversation, the next year my business began falling apart. As often happens in these cases, my behavior changed in subtle ways I wasn't immediately aware of. For instance, I became slightly less responsive to my clients and began spending more than I previously had. In small ways that quickly added up, I was making decisions that lessened my chances of success. Before long, my external circumstances began to reflect these decisions; several projects I needed fell through, and other clients stopped paying me. And within 12 months of that phone call with my friend, I had accumulated massive personal debt. The upside of my financial distress was that I could commiserate with my friends again. We were all in the same boat, and no one had reason to be jealous of me.

When I discovered tapping years later, I realized what had happened and used tapping to overcome my unconscious mind's fear of losing friends as a result of financial success. Since then, my relationship with success and money has been transformed, along with my sense of what's possible for anyone who's willing to see and challenge their most basic beliefs, whether it's about money, pain, love, or something else.

My story is just one example of how the unconscious mind works. Because it's so skilled at protecting you, it is very good at hiding emotions, beliefs, and memories from you that you may need to face before pain relief is possible. Throughout this chapter, we'll explore ways that your unconscious mind may be holding on to pain, thus sabotaging your pain-relief efforts.

When We Become the Pain

Jesi had been in chronic pain since she was 14 years old. Now almost 40, she'd lived with fibromyalgia for so long that she could barely remember what it was like to be pain-free. After attending my pain-relief event and tapping through several traumatic childhood memories, she'd experienced a 30 to 40 percent reduction in pain. Several months had passed since the event, however, and she could now feel her pain returning. "Just as life has progressed, the pain is back up . . . not back to where it was before the event, but it's back up to the point where it's interfering with my life again," she explained. "Knowing where to go next [with my tapping] is really difficult for me . . . I just want pain relief, and I'm willing to do whatever I need to do to get it. I really believe in this process."

As she was sharing this at the start of our session, she could feel a crunching pain in her jaw, as well as pain in her wrist, hands, shoulders, and the backs of her thighs. To begin, I asked Jesi to tap through the points at her own pace while imagining herself pain-free.

She spoke out loud and shared what that vision was: "Just more of who I am and what I do already, just more of it. Less downtime, fewer interruptions, fewer cancellations of lessons, and more of doing what I love to do."

When Jesi's pain had begun at age 14, the pain had been her way of seeking comfort and relief from the emotional pain she felt at school and at home. That didn't resonate with her any longer, however. With a family and career she loves, she's created a very happy life for herself. When she's in pain now, she loses out on the things and people she values most—her husband, her daughter, and the work she loves to do. She no longer needs the pain as an excuse to hide.

"Do you think your body got the memo?" I asked.

In other words, was her unconscious mind sending opposing messages to her body? Until we used tapping to explore her relationship with pain and pain relief, she didn't realize how deeply ingrained her pattern of pain had become.

I led Jesi through several rounds of tapping on feeling safe without the pain, wanting to send her unconscious mind and her body the message that it no longer needed to use pain to protect her. She was surrounded by people who loved her and a career that brought her tremendous joy and fulfillment.

As we tapped, the pain began to move, which suggested that we were on the right track. She also began to sweat. She felt feverish, which was unusual. While tapping, she also had several aha! moments around how ingrained pain had become in her identity and her life. Since she had never lived as an adult without pain, a pain-free vision of herself and her life was unknown to her. It made sense that her unconscious mind perceived the idea as dangerous and held on to her pain as a result. To become pain-free, Jesi needed to reinvent herself as someone who didn't have chronic pain.

By the end of our 45-minute session, the pain in Jesi's jaw, her wrists, and the backs of her thighs had disappeared. Her shoulder pain had moved into the middle of her back and had gone from an 8 out of 10 down to a 5 out of 10. Given how much pain relief Jesi had gotten from our session, I recommended that she continue to focus her tapping on feeling safe letting go of the pain. Through tapping, she also needed to create a pain-free vision of her life that didn't make her sweat, literally or figuratively.

Because pain quickly takes over your life, over time it can begin to determine how you feel, then what you do. Eventually, pain can become *who* you are. Do you identify yourself—who you are and who you can be—as someone with pain? I often hear people say they're a "different person" when they're in pain. It would be impossible not to act and feel differently when you're in pain. Over time, however, the "different person" you become with the pain can begin to dominate your identity, making it hard for other parts of yourself and your life to shine through.

• •

Because pain quickly takes over your life, over time it can begin to determine how you feel, then what you do. Eventually, pain can become who you are . . . Do you identify yourself—who you are and who you can be—as someone with pain?

• •

Has Pain Become Part of Who You Are?

With your journal in hand, take a moment now to think, *Who would I be without this pain?* Write down everything that comes to mind. If nothing comes up, try tapping through the points while asking yourself that question.

Some of the beliefs clients often discover when they do this exercise are:

- I don't know who I am without this pain.
- My pain takes up all my time.
- I won't know what to expect if this changes.
- Change means that more bad things will happen.
- If I don't have pain, I'll have to _____.

To begin clearing these beliefs, let's do some tapping on them now. Remember, this is general tapping on a global belief. As ideas, memories, and more specific things come up, tap on them individually.

Before tapping, say out loud, "I don't know who I'll be without this pain." How true does that feel on a 0-to-10 scale? Also notice your pain and give it a number. Write these both down in your journal. Now start tapping:

Karate Chop: Even though I don't know who I'll be without this pain, I still choose to accept myself.

Karate Chop: Even though this pain has been my identity, I still choose to accept myself and I still choose to release this pain.

Karate Chop: Even though this pain has been with me for so long, and I don't know what I would do with myself without it, I still choose to accept myself and I still choose to release this pain.

Eyebrow: This pain has become a big part of my life.

Side of Eye: I've been living around this pain for a long time now.

Under Eye: I expect to have this pain . . .

Under Nose: A part of me needs this pain . . .

Chin: Who will I be without this pain . . .

Collarbone: Will I be able to handle it all . . .

Under Arm: What if it's all too much . . .

Top of Head: I can't let go of this pain.

Eyebrow: What if I let go of this pain and I'm still not happy . . .

Side of Eye: I want to want to let go of this pain . . .

Under Eye: But I'm not sure how.

Under Nose: I'm not sure I can.

Chin: Don't I need this pain to keep me safe . . .

Collarbone: This pain is a part of my life.

Under Arm: This pain makes me feel special.

Top of Head: I don't know how to handle life without this pain.

Take a few deep breaths and, once again, say out loud, "I don't know who I'll be without this pain." How true does that feel on a 0-to-10 scale now? Has your pain shifted at all? Write down any changes in your journal. Keep tapping on the "negative" until it's a 5 or lower, and then move on to the positive rounds.

Positive Round

Eyebrow: This pain is just a time in my life . . .

Side of Eye: It is not who I am.

Under Eye: I choose to remember that I am many things.

Under Nose: There is a new chapter to my life . . .

Chin: I am more than I have given myself credit for.

Collarbone: I look forward to making new discoveries . . .

Under Arm: About myself and my life.

Top of Head: I can be free from pain and be safe to be me.

Eyebrow: I don't need this pain to define me.

Side of Eye: It is not who I am.

Under Eye: I know that I am many things . . .

Under Nose: And I can move forward into a new chapter in my life . . .

Chin: A chapter without pain . . .

Collarbone: And I can change what isn't working . . .

Under Arm: And enjoy what is working in my body and my life . . .

Top of Head: I can be free from pain and feel safe being pain-free.

What Pain Relief Brings

Pain relief may seem like the only thing you want, but when you drill down into what that would mean for you in your life, you may discover relationships or parts of your life you'd rather not face. Unlike Jesi, with her fear of the unknown, Kimi realized in our first session that getting better for her meant facing a known life she didn't like. After she'd invested years in a successful career as a banker, the neck pain from her frozen shoulder, or Thoracic Outlet Syndrome, had gotten so bad that she could no longer work. She'd seen multiple doctors and tried cortisone shots, but nothing had worked. Eventually, she'd had to quit her job and go on disability. More recently, she'd also undergone carpal tunnel surgery.

When I asked Kimi what had been happening in her life when the pain first began, she said that she'd been working at the Beverly Hills branch of a London-based bank. The working atmosphere there was toxic. At the time, the bank was downsizing, and her boss was being investigated for financial misconduct. As one of the few women in a male-dominated industry, she felt her ideas were been ignored, even though she was one of the most experienced bankers in the office.

When I asked Kimi to imagine herself pain-free, off disability, and returning to work, she felt nauseous. "I still don't know what I want to do when I grow up," she explained. After several rounds of tapping on her anxiety about returning to work, the nausea was replaced by a different sensation. "I can feel it in my gut. It's like a dark hole in my gut," she shared. The emotion in that dark hole was fear.

After several rounds of tapping, her fear went away, and she could feel a pressing pain moving up the right side of her neck, going toward her throat.

"The pressing pain is about not using my voice," she said.

At work, she tended to be quiet and not express her feelings or ideas. In the financial services industry, she explained, women's ideas are looked down on.

"They try all the men's ideas, and then turn and ask you [the woman in the room] for your ideas, and when you tell them, they sarcastically say, 'Oh, that's a great idea.'"

I asked if that had made her angry.

"I've worked through a lot of anger at men," she explained, "but at this point, I've accepted that women aren't heard. We aren't supposed to speak up. I'm just waiting for things to change."

Sensing that Kimi had stuffed down more anger toward men than she realized, I led her through several rounds of tapping on it.

"Even though I have all this anger in my body, I can think of all these times when things weren't right, and I didn't say anything . . . I swallowed it down . . . all this anger in my body . . . the way they treated me wasn't right . . . all those times when I wanted to say something . . . but I swallowed it down . . . and if I let go of this pain . . . I have to go back to work . . . and I don't want to go back to that . . . it's safe to feel this rage . . . I have a right to feel it . . . and I choose to let it go . . . releasing this anger from my body now."

When we were done, I asked her how the tapping had felt. "Empowering," she replied. The pain in her throat and under her armpit had both gone from a 6 out of 10 down to a 3 out of 10. The pain in her throat had also moved higher up and from the side of her throat to the back of her throat, which had never happened before.

To test her results, I asked her again to imagine being pain-free and returning to work. "I feel heaviness in my heart because going back to work in financial services is not my calling," she explained. We did more tapping on the remainder of her pain, and on the remaining rage she'd felt at how men had treated her, sending her body and unconscious mind the message that it's safe to feel "big" emotions like anger and rage.

Afterward, I asked Kimi to share one memory that represents how she was treated at the office.

"Being the senior banker in my office, and not having a voice, and just having to sit back and let everyone decide what will happen . . . There was one man, he was from France, who would veto or undermine everything I said . . . making everything feel like a power struggle . . . [and me] feeling powerless, and not being able to do anything but feel enraged, having no one to talk to, the only woman there, just being all alone and feeling enraged," she shared as memories flashed through her mind.

I asked her to imagine sitting there feeling powerless and being enraged. "Where do you feel it in your body?" I asked.

"In my heart," she replied.

To give Kimi a chance to claim her voice, I then asked her to run her memory of just sitting there, but this time imagining that she said something different.

"Feel fear and anxiety when you're about to, but still say it," I instructed her.

"You don't know anything," she said, laughing.

"Feel how good it feels to say that," I guided her. "See yourself as strong and confident, knowing what you're talking about."

She then proceeded to say what she'd wanted to say for many years. "Everything that you're suggesting doesn't make sense in our society and our culture, and we need a different approach to be successful," she said, envisioning herself speaking to that former colleague from France whom she felt had always tried to silence and undermine her.

By the end of our session, Kimi realized that pain was her body's way of allowing her to avoid returning to the hostile, suffocating environment she'd experienced at work. The rage she felt as a result of that working environment was too much to face, so her body had created the pain to distract her. Since her pain had lowered and moved up into her throat, she was able to cancel an appointment to get muscle blocker shots in her neck. Instead, she would spend that time researching new career options for the future.

"Sometimes it takes a lot of digging," I shared as we were finishing our session. "But now you know you can do this. So just buckle down and in a couple of days, the pain could all be gone. You want to run that picture of you going back to work, and feel that anxiety and feel that anger, because it's helping you connect with that rage. What you'll find as you tap through these emotions and clear them is that other ideas will come up, so the whole thing starts becoming a lot more positive. Right now, the pain going away has a big downside for you. You've got to get to the point where you can imagine the pain going away, and there's a huge upside because you've figured out what you want to do next . . . If you can't create a positive picture of your pain going away and that being a good thing, then the pain is going to hang on. We've just gotten great results in forty-five minutes, so see if you can commit to spending forty-five minutes a day on tapping through these issues."

Several days later, Kimi sent me an e-mail updating me on her progress. After our session, her pain had decreased so dramatically that she'd been able to go off all medication. She had also begun training for a new position in mind–body healing and was feeling energized and excited about her future. While tapping, she'd also identified several childhood traumas that were additional sources of her rage against men, and she was working through those as well.

"Eternally grateful," she wrote. "Big fan [of tapping]. Huge supporter of EFT. And I still tap whenever I have time."

What's the Downside of Pain Relief?

Grab your journal and a pen. Then close your eyes and imagine that your pain is gone. Notice how great your body feels. For the first time in a long time, there is no pain. Next, ask yourself, *What's the downside of my pain going away?*

Do you have to return to a job you hate? Do you lose the excuse to avoid difficult and/or new relationships? What parts of yourself or your life will you have to face when the pain is gone?

In your journal, write down anything and everything that comes to mind. If you can't come up with any, make something up. Write down issues other people might have to face if they got rid of the pain.

When I led the audience at one of my pain-relief events through this journaling exercise and asked who wanted to share what they'd discovered, a sea of hands went up. Here are a few of the discoveries people shared:

"I already feel overwhelmed with everything I have to do. If I didn't have the pain, I'd have even less time for myself, and I always feel guilty taking time for myself because there's just so much to do."

"I've been taking photography classes and really trying to hone that skill. And if I didn't have the pain, my husband would expect me to do more with that, and I have a big fear of failure, but also of success."

"Before I had pain, I was doing so much, but it never felt like enough. If I didn't have the pain, it would be great, but at the same time, I would have no limitation, and that old feeling would come back."

"Without the pain, I would have to say no to people, and no isn't in my vocabulary."

"One of the things that I would really miss is my husband doing my hair, because with the pain, I can't hold the hair dryer up."

"I wouldn't be special anymore. People wouldn't open the door for me anymore. I've always had the feeling that only blond, slim people get that special treatment, and I've always been the athletic, self-sufficient one."

"I was a commercial pilot, and I wasn't feeling very confident in that job, and if the pain goes away, then I have to decide if I want to continue being a commercial pilot or if I want to voluntarily give up that role."

"The pain allows me an excuse to not find another permanent relationship because the last one was very hard for me, and with the limitations of my illness, I have made that an excuse, so I don't have to go and find another relationship. It's easier to stay alone."

Do any of these or similar themes resonate with you? If so, add them to your journal.

When you're ready, let's do some tapping on feeling safe without the pain. Before tapping, say out loud, "It's not safe to let go of this pain." How true does it feel on a 0-to-10 scale? Give your pain a separate number and write both in your journal. As you tap, notice what other ideas, memories, events, and emotions come up regarding this belief and the pain. Tap on those specifically as you go along.

Karate Chop: Even though a part of me is afraid to let go of this pain, I still choose to accept myself.

Karate Chop: Even though I'm not sure if I can feel safe without this pain, I accept myself and these feelings.

Karate Chop: Even though this pain is helping me somehow, I still choose to accept myself and I still choose to release this pain.

Eyebrow: A part of me is afraid to let go of this pain . . .

Side of Eye: Some part of me still needs this pain.

Under Eye: I don't know how to keep myself safe without this pain . . .

Under Nose: I've had this pain for so long.

Chin: I'm not sure what will change if I don't have it.

Collarbone: What if there are changes I can't handle . . .

Under Arm: This pain is familiar . . .

Top of Head: I know what to expect.

Eyebrow: This pain keeps me hidden.

Side of Eye: This pain lets me rest.

Under Eye: This pain lets me say no.

Under Nose: This pain keeps some people away.

Chin: This pain keeps some people close . . .

Collarbone: This pain gets their attention . . .

Under Arm: This pain gets my attention.

Top of Head: How will I be safe when I no longer have this pain . . .

Check in with yourself. If being pain-free still seems unsafe, keep tapping on the "negative" until it's a 5 or lower before moving on to the positive. Also take a moment to notice if your pain has shifted.

Positive Round

Eyebrow: I am ready to release this pain.

Side of Eye: I can find ways to take care of myself.

Under Eye: I choose to find ways to protect me.

Under Nose: I can find ways to say no.

Chin: I am stronger than I give myself credit for.

Collarbone: I remember that I am resourceful . . .

Under Arm: That I have a voice and that I matter.

Top of Head: I can release this pain and be safe.

Take a deep breath. Check back in with your original statement, "It's not safe to let go of this pain," and see how true it feels now on a 0-to-10 scale. Keep tapping until it's a 3 or lower, or until you get the relief you desire. Notice also if your pain has shifted.

Creating Healthy Boundaries

As we explore the upsides to pain and the downsides to pain relief, there's a pattern we see on both sides of the issue, and that's the absence of healthy boundaries. When we set healthy boundaries, we can take care of ourselves. As a result, the unconscious mind no longer needs to create chronic pain to divert our attention away from the parts of ourselves or our lives that feel unsafe. The healthy boundaries basically do that work before the unconscious mind gets involved. When we don't set boundaries, however, we allow people to do and say things that feel unsafe, and then stuff down the emotions we feel in response. As we've seen, over time those repressed emotions can then contribute to chronic pain.

Madison had always struggled with creating healthy boundaries, especially with friends who didn't always support her and often crossed boundaries she didn't know how to keep. For years her migraines had allowed her to avoid those friends. The pain had given her a valid reason to turn down social invitations that made her uncomfortable.

ASK YOURSELF: How do you feel about saying no? Do you feel as though you have the right to say no to people and situations in your life that make you uncomfortable in some way? If not, do some tapping on your resistance to saying no.

When I asked Madison to imagine getting better, she quickly began to feel overwhelmed. While on one level, she wanted nothing more than pain relief, she also felt hesitant about what life would be like without the pain. As much as she wanted relief from her migraine pain, getting better also felt stressful. Without the pain, she wouldn't have an easy excuse to avoid friends. She would need to learn to say no instead, and that might make her friends mad. Even worse, she might end up completely alone, without any friends at all.

After working together over several weeks, tapping through her fear and other emotions, Madison began to set healthy boundaries with friends. Instead of saying yes to every invitation, she checked in with herself and responded according to what she needed and wanted to do instead. The more Madison did this, the less migraine pain she experienced, until finally her pain disappeared altogether. Because she had actively removed the need for pain as an excuse to avoid friends, her unconscious mind got the message that Madison could use healthy boundaries to take care of herself without the pain.

• •

When we set healthy boundaries, we can take care of ourselves. As a result, the unconscious mind no longer needs to create chronic pain to divert our attention away from the parts of ourselves or our lives that feel unsafe.

• •

Where Do You Need to Set Boundaries?

Often we don't realize where in our lives we're not setting healthy boundaries. Dr. Brené Brown, *New York Times* best-selling author of *The Gifts of Imperfection*, has an exercise for figuring that out. She calls it a "resentment journal."

Take a moment now to write your own resentment journal. Make a list of memories and situations you feel resentful about. Also include events that caused you discomfort, which is another common reaction to someone crossing your boundary.

When you're done writing your resentment journal, pick the event that brings up the most resentment and give your resentment a number from 0 to 10. Then tap on it.

Once your resentment is a 3 or lower, imagine what kind of boundary you could set to avoid the circumstances that caused you to feel resentful. Could you say no instead of yes? Could you ask for help instead of trying to manage things by yourself? Could you voice your feelings when someone questions the validity of your pain and/or illness?

While tapping through the points, imagine being in that situation again, but this time, set a boundary that would allow you to feel safe. Say what you wanted to say but didn't; do what you wish you'd done. Notice any emotions that come up when you imagine setting those boundaries and let yourself feel them as you're tapping. Keep tapping until the event or memory loses its emotional charge.

Use this process to clear all the events listed in your resentment journal. If your list is long, commit to tapping through one or two per day. You'll be amazed by how much you can clear in a relatively short time.

As you begin to clear the events in your resentment journal, you'll also get a better handle on what boundaries you need to establish.

How to Create Healthy Boundaries

There are many ways to create healthy boundaries, for example, saying no when you've always said yes, speaking up when you've always been quiet, not sharing parts of yourself or your life with people who aren't supportive. For most of us, it's like learning a new skill, which is usually awkward and uncomfortable at first. It can also be scary because we fear we'll damage or lose important relationships.

The first step is to train your unconscious brain that it's safe for you to create healthy boundaries. To begin, start small and pick a situation that doesn't feel threatening or where you have little to lose by creating a boundary. It could be as simple as letting a phone call from an unsupportive friend or family member go to voice mail.

Keep that picture in your mind and let yourself feel any emotions you feel around setting the boundary. Now let's do some tapping on it being safe to create that boundary.

When you think about setting that boundary, how unsafe does it feel? Give it a number on a scale of 0 to 10. Also notice how your pain feels and give your pain its own number. Write these both in your journal and then start tapping:

Karate Chop: Even though I'm not sure how to set boundaries, to stick up for myself, I accept myself and I'm open to learning.

Karate Chop: Even though I never learned to set boundaries, I still accept myself and I'm willing to learn.

Karate Chop: Even though it's not comfortable for me to think about setting boundaries, to say what I want, I accept all of me and maybe I can give it a try.

Eyebrow: I don't know how to set boundaries.

Side of Eye: I find it hard to stick up for myself.

Under Eye: If I set a boundary, they will be mad at me . . .

Under Nose: I know I would feel uncomfortable having that conversation.

Chin: They wouldn't like it.

Collarbone: I'm afraid of their reaction to me speaking my mind . . .

Under Arm: I'm not good at speaking my mind . . .

Top of Head: I'm not good at asking for what I want.

Eyebrow: I'm scared to set boundaries . . .

Side of Eye: I'm scared about how they'll react . . .

Under Eye: I'm scared about what they'll say to me . . .

Under Nose: I don't feel like I can set boundaries.

Chin: They won't like it.

Collarbone: Setting boundaries will just cause more problems . . .

Under Arm: Setting boundaries will just make my life more difficult . . .

Top of Head: I'm so scared to set boundaries, but I also know I really need to.

Check in with yourself and notice how you're feeling about setting the boundary. Give it a number on a scale of 0 to 10. Keep tapping on the "negative" until the intensity is a 5 or lower and then switch to some positive rounds. Also notice any shifts in your pain. Remember, these scripts are just here for guidance and to get you started. Feel free to use your own language, speak your own truth, and so forth.

Positive Round

Eyebrow: I don't feel comfortable asking for what I want . . .

Side of Eye: I'm not sure I have the right to ask for what I want.

Under Eye: But what if I could . . .

Under Nose: Maybe this is something I could try . . .

Chin: Find a small step where I could practice . . .

Collarbone: I can find safe people to start with.

Under Arm: I can get in touch with what I want.

Top of Head: I can be excited to start this journey.

Eyebrow: I deserve to be heard.

Side of Eye: I can know what I want.

Under Eye: I can start to ask for what I want.

Under Nose: I choose to be open to setting boundaries.

Chin: When I respect my feelings . . .

Collarbone: And ask for what I need . . .

Under Arm: I'm showing myself respect.

Top of Head: I'm honoring who I am.

Check in with yourself and notice how you're feeling about setting the boundary. Give it a number on a scale of 0 to 10. Keep tapping until you feel ready to take action on setting a boundary.

How Pain Impacts Relationships

Sometimes, even after we set healthy boundaries, people cross them, and we need to look more closely at our relationships. Many people find that their relationships suffer because of their chronic pain. They feel misunderstood, judged, and isolated because of their pain, and they don't know how to create healthy boundaries that would improve their experience within relationships.

Hana knew this problem well. Most of her relationships had been negatively impacted by her chronic pain and other health issues. Over the years, Hana's parents had repeatedly questioned her pain and illness in subtle and overt ways, often insisting that she didn't need a wheelchair in restaurants when she felt she did. There was also the time her mom refused Hana her crutches, and the other time when her mom had failed to lower Hana's medical toilet seat, even after Hana had specifically asked her to, causing her to nearly get stuck on the toilet shortly after undergoing surgery.

More recently, a trusted friend had asked Hana about her health, and then delivered a short lecture on the importance of physical therapy. Even her surgeon seemed skeptical about the health issues she experienced as a result of her connective tissue disease.

Over and over again, people had made Hana feel as if she wasn't doing enough to better her health and get rid of her pain, when in fact researching her conditions and taking care of her pain and her disease consumed most of Hana's time and energy. When I asked her how she felt when she thought of these events, she replied that they made her feel "kind of pissed off." Although she was aware of her anger, she didn't feel that she could express it, or say much of anything, without risking her most important relationships.

Dealing with Toxic Relationships: When Boundaries Won't Stick

When people repeatedly cross your boundaries, even after you've clearly communicated them, you may need to consider whether you're in a toxic relationship. If the emotional residue of a toxic relationship is related to your pain, you may not be able to experience pain relief until you take the necessary steps to distance yourself from that relationship. If you find yourself in this situation, get support to find ways to manage or remove yourself from a toxic relationship.

It's a common experience. As one woman at a live event expressed, "One of my biggest fears is going back home and having my friends question me about my experience here and getting the same response I always get, which is like, when are you going to stop all this nonsense? It's discouraging."

Another shared, "I'm afraid that tapping won't work for me, and if it doesn't, I'll have to explain another wild scheme to my friends. I feel silly, and then they tell me to stop the woo-woo. They tell me to just buck up," she explained.

When we're unable to set healthy boundaries in these kinds of situations, responses like these can send the unconscious mind running for cover, eager to create more pain to distract us from people and situations in our lives that don't feel safe.

Four Tips for Creating Healthy Boundaries

As you begin to create healthy boundaries for yourself, keep in mind these simple but powerful tips, which were provided by Donna M. White, LPCI, CACP, on Psych Central:

1. **Get clear on the boundary you need to set.** Use tapping to get in touch with where your boundaries lie with different people and in different situations. It's normal for them to vary from one person to the next, so don't worry if your boundaries aren't consistent from one relationship to another. The goal is to get clear on where your boundaries are with different people and in different situations.

2. **Be firm when you set your boundary.** To explain why you're creating a boundary, you may want to share your feelings or experience, but then be firm about the boundary you're setting. Don't let yourself be talked out of setting your boundary.

3. **Remember you're not responsible for someone else's response.** You're setting boundaries for yourself and your own well-being, which means you can't be responsible for other people's reactions. Other people's reactions are not your responsibility. You need to focus on taking care of yourself so that your unconscious mind doesn't hold on to chronic pain in order to protect you from the people and situations where your boundaries get crossed.

4. **Remember that it's a process.** Learning to create healthy boundaries is a process, so be gentle with yourself and know that it may take time to learn how to create healthy boundaries. Get support, seek out feedback, and be open to new and better ways of approaching the process.

A Tapping Process for Clearing Resentment and Setting Boundaries

Here's a tapping process that can help you clear resentment from past attempts to create boundaries and set healthy new boundaries with people now.

Imagine five different people in your life who have hurt you or crossed your boundary in some way. Pick one to start and imagine them standing in front of you. If you could tell them anything or ask them anything about how you felt or what happened between you, what would it be? Imagine yourself doing that—what feelings come up? Anger, hurt, fear, guilt?

This is what gets in the way of setting the boundary and where tapping comes in. Tap through all the feelings that come up, allowing yourself time to imagine that person's reaction and then notice the next set of feelings that rise to the surface.

Ask yourself, *Where else have I felt this way? What does this feeling remind me of?*

Tap on those other events as they present themselves. If nothing comes up, that's okay as well; just continue tapping for the feelings that were coming up when you were expressing your thoughts and feelings to the person you imagined.

Check in with that image again. When you see yourself in front of that person, how does it feel now? Continue to tap around the remaining feelings that might come up in that conversation. Imagine how they might react to your request—notice if there are feelings coming up for you. When you find them, tap on those feelings. This step could take some time—or it could take only a few minutes. Remember, you are doing this for you, so if it takes a little time to go through the process, it's worth it because you're worth it. The more time you spend working through the different scenarios, the more natural it will feel when you do ask for what you need or want.

Once you've walked through the process for your imaginary person number one, do the same for the next person on your list. Notice if the next person was easier, or if different feelings came up. You might find that the process moves quickly with some people while other people on your list are more challenging. Once you become good at setting boundaries and speaking up for what you want, you'll still find people who present more of a challenge, but think of all the practice you'll have gotten doing this exercise!

Audio Bonus: If you'd like to explore the upside and downside of pain relief, as well as some powerful positive tapping on a future without pain, join me in a bonus free tapping meditation here: thetappingsolution.com/painbookresources.

CHAPTER 9

CREATING A NEW RELATIONSHIP WITH YOURSELF, YOUR BODY, AND YOUR LIFE

Now that we've looked at, and hopefully cleared, the internal blocks to pain relief, it's a good time to step back and take a look at the overall relationship with yourself, your body, and your life. This will help you build a solid foundation for long-lasting pain relief, as well as overall health and wellness.

The Key to Lasting Pain Relief

It was the final day of a pain-relief event and several audience members raised their hands to share experiences from the night before.

"What happens with me is that I wake up in the middle of the night with excruciating cramps," one woman began. "And it happened again last night. My foot was throbbing, and at first I thought, maybe [tapping] is just not working for me, maybe I'm not working hard enough. But then I remembered you saying it's not just about the pain, that it's really about how we feel about ourselves, so I stopped and asked myself, how do I feel about myself? And I thought, I feel so much better about myself. And maybe that's the journey I have ahead of me. Maybe I need to feel better about myself, accept myself, love myself more . . . and maybe that's the key."

"If you get to pick between loving and accepting yourself or getting rid of the pain," I responded, "go for loving and accepting yourself. I know the pain sucks, I know it really, really sucks, but go toward self-love and self-acceptance because everything builds from there."

Let me say that again.

Once you've cleared the underlying issues of your pain and as you continue to clear them, the key is to focus on self-acceptance and self-love, because together they create the foundation for lasting pain relief, as well as overall health and wellness.

. . . .

If you get to pick between loving and accepting yourself or getting rid of the pain, go for loving and accepting yourself. I know the pain sucks, I know it really, really sucks, but go toward self-love and self-acceptance because everything builds from there.

. . . .

Relearning to Love and Accept Yourself

When pain has been a constant for so long, the frustration and hopelessness it creates gradually eat away at self-esteem and often feed into old patterns of beating up on ourselves. Brianna began to see this in herself during our third session to address the pain she was feeling in her shoulders.

"Being in pain," she shared, "it's hard to get yourself in a better-feeling place . . . I fully understand concepts like positive thinking, but still, it's a constant battle. It's like, how do you turn it off when it feels like the body is falling apart? I like what you said, Nick, about recognizing what is working in my body, because there *is* a lot in my body that is working. But trying to figure out if I'm improving or getting worse is kind of a preoccupation with my physical state from one day to the next. And my physical state sometimes leads to frustration and anger. I get that 'why me?' feeling. When is this going to end? And there's a part of me that knows this is a process, and it's not going to turn off overnight. So it's a roller coaster for me. I have good days when I think, I can do this; I can heal."

After a slight pause, she continued: "And then there are days when I'm in that pit of darkness, when I feel like I'm being punished. I look around me, and certainly friends have other issues, but they're not struggling with their health the way I am. And I don't like the quality of my life. I'm constantly going back and forth between hope, frustration, and anger. I'm just all over the place."

At the start of our session, the pain in Brianna's shoulders was an 8 out of 10. Each time she tapped, her pain would subside the next day but then return with a vengeance soon afterward. After tapping on various issues for a few weeks, she was beginning to wonder whether permanent pain relief would ever happen for her. Even when she felt good, she didn't feel as if she could trust her body to hold on to that good feeling. The pain would return, regardless.

"Sometimes it's overwhelming, and I just give up. I have this feeling of indifference. I don't like it, but I just get to a point where I don't care anymore. It's just like, this is what it is; this is all that's possible for me."

To begin clearing her feelings of hopelessness, I led Brianna through multiple rounds of tapping on her frustration and her mistrust of her body. As her pain began to decrease, I began to focus our tapping on cultivating self-acceptance and self-love.

"I've been so hard on myself . . . I've been beating up on myself . . . And now I can be kinder to myself . . . I can approve of my body as it is . . . I can accept my body as it is . . . I accept myself as I am . . . " I guided her through additional tapping rounds.

When we were done, she commented on how much the idea of beating up on herself resonated with her.

"A lightbulb went off. It was like, yeah, I have been beating myself up and my body feels beaten. [Beating myself up] is a comfortable place, a familiar place . . . It's like a groove I keep falling into, as opposed to being loving, nurturing, and patient with myself. That's a big one," she said.

I suggested that she visualize physically beating on her own body every time she caught herself mentally beating up on herself. "Because essentially, that's what you're doing," I explained. "If you hit your back and neck and shoulders a hundred times a day, it would start to hurt."

Again and again, I've seen pain clients who have spent so many years being hard on themselves that it's become second nature. Until I point it out, they often don't recognize how often they mentally beat themselves up. This pattern is a critical one to address and clear through tapping.

As you begin looking at turning negative, self-critical thoughts into positive, self-loving thoughts, it's important to understand that it's a process. Few of us go from beating up on ourselves to loving and accepting ourselves overnight, or in a single tapping session. It takes time to relearn how to treat ourselves with love, consideration, and respect.

We also need to remember that our goal is not necessarily to think only positive thoughts. I don't know anyone who can do that. It's a process of learning to have more positive thoughts, so over time, they begin to outweigh the negative ones.

ASK YOURSELF: What negative thoughts keep running through my head? When I make a mistake, do I forgive myself or continue harping on my mistake? Do I blame myself for other people's unhappiness or misfortune? Do I feel like I'm somehow not enough? Do I look in the mirror and immediately criticize what I see?

Few of us go from beating up on ourselves to loving and accepting ourselves overnight, or in a single tapping session. It takes time to relearn how to treat ourselves with love, consideration, and respect.

Begin to notice how you treat yourself on a daily basis and make notes in your journal of what you discover. Be sure to tap through these thought patterns. Until you clear the emotions and beliefs behind these thoughts, they will continue to interfere with your health and well-being.

Trust the Process More Than You Trust the Fear

I often hear from clients about what they used to do before they had chronic pain. They loved to take long walks. They loved to cook. They biked to work every day. They loved to garden on the weekends. They spent time painting, making music, swimming, playing with their kids. Those activities made them feel good. They were simple ways of taking care of themselves, of expressing self-love and self-acceptance.

Before her chronic neck pain, Tara's self-care had always centered around yoga. She had loved yoga and how it made her feel physically, emotionally, and mentally. Since her neck pain started, though, she had avoided yoga and all movements that involved her neck, upper back, and shoulders. Every time she tried using those muscles, she would wake up the following day with an excruciating migraine.

Years after being in multiple car accidents and also being assaulted, Tara was diagnosed with severe whiplash that had turned into cervical stenosis, "which meant I had the neck of an eighty-nine-year-old woman in my early thirties," she explained. Seven years after her diagnosis, her neck had grown so weak that she had been unable to hold it upright. The weight of her head had become more than her neck could bear. In hopes of regaining strength and movement, she underwent a rare and extreme surgical procedure, a seven-level cervical laminectomy in which they'd removed much of the bone from the back of her cervical spinal column.

Since the surgery, Tara and her husband had spent $100,000 on physical therapy, and while she had regained the mobility to roll her head and do yoga, each time she tried, she would wake up the following day with that same excruciating migraine. As a result, she began to avoid yoga again. As much as she missed it— and other activities that involved her neck, shoulders, and arms—it wasn't worth the pain.

After hearing her story, I started our session by asking Tara what her neck felt like. "I feel like there are all these tears in my neck," she replied. After multiple rounds of tapping on the tears in her neck, and the emotions behind those tears, I asked her to roll her neck from side to side. Sure that she would get a migraine the following day, Tara panicked but agreed to do it anyway. Once she had rolled her neck around in a complete circle, I asked her to do her favorite yoga pose.

That idea scared her so much that she began to cry. "When you asked me to do that," she later told me, "I was sure you didn't understand my condition."

Determined to move forward, though, she nonetheless got into her favorite yoga pose, which is called warrior pose.

To Tara's shock and amazement, she woke up the next morning feeling fine. "There was no pain, no migraine," she recalled when we spoke again several months later. "And now when people ask me about my neck, I'm like, oh, it's fine. I don't even think about my neck any more. I forget it used to be a problem," she shared. "It's pretty exciting! My life is not restricted the way it used to be."

Before our one tapping session, she explained, "My whole life was about what I couldn't do. My life became super, super small, and I absolutely was depressed. It was like my body was taken away. I couldn't take the garbage out, couldn't lift the laundry. The thing with that was feeling so dependent at such a young age. It squashed the independence in me." Later she told me, "My neck and the migraines were a life-stopping situation. It wasn't a roadblock. It was more like the street was permanently closed, but tapping on my neck with you that day did something internally, emotionally with me. It was like, ta-da! The road is now open."

During that tapping session, Tara's entire life turned around. Instead of just existing, she once again began living her life. Looking back on herself and her life before our session, she added, "If I could give advice to someone with chronic pain like I had, I'd say, trust the process more than you trust the fear."

What Would You Do If the Pain Vanished?

Sometimes the best thing you can do is to stop focusing on the pain and take time to do things that make you feel good. That seems impossible when the pain won't go away, or seems sure to return, but by doing things that make you feel good, you're practicing and expressing the self-love and self-acceptance that are the basis of lasting pain relief and overall health and wellness.

• •

Sometimes the best thing you can do is to stop focusing on the pain and take time to do things that make you feel good . . . To move toward a pain-free future, you will need to begin opening up to new possibilities—new ways of relating to your body, your life, and yourself.

• •

To move toward a pain-free future, you will need to begin opening up to new possibilities—new ways of relating to your body, your life, and yourself. Take a moment now to get your journal and a pen or pencil. Then ask yourself, *What would I do if I had no pain?* List anything and everything that comes to mind, from doing the laundry to working in your garden, traveling around the world, going for a run, playing with your children, or pursuing a new career. Whatever comes to mind, write it down. Keep this list; we'll be coming back to it later.

A Doctor Taps Away His Chronic Knee and Shoulder Pain

While teaching tapping to physicians attending a conference an integrative health for pain management, Lori Leyden, Ph.D., the director of The Tapping Solution Foundation, worked with one physician who had been experiencing chronic knee and shoulder pain for several years. During a group tapping session the doctor was shocked to find that his pain went from a 7 out of 10 down to a 4 out of 10.

The next day the doctor did a private session with Lori. As they were tapping, he indicated that his pain continued to be better since tapping the day before; it was still a 4 out of 10. During their session, he also voiced his limiting belief that the pain prevented him from playing competitive tennis. As they were tapping, he also connected his pain to the trauma of watching his father wither away from a stroke for four years because of poor medical care, as well as his grief and sadness over having lost 12 of his 14 family members over the years.

By then end of the session, his range of motion had improved significantly and his pain had gone down to a 1 out of 10, which he was thrilled about! When Lori asked about his concern about playing competitive tennis, he said it didn't matter because there were so many other things he could do. He also indicated that he could be such a better caregiver to his patients because it now felt safe to be vulnerable.

The pain relief he got from tapping allowed him to create a new relationship with his body and discover hidden benefits that would make him a better caregiver.

When Pain Runs Your Life

Over time pain often takes over more than the body. It disrupts other parts of life as well. After our session, Tara could see how this had played out in her life. Once her chronic neck pain had taken over her body, depression set in, and from there, her entire life seemed to spiral downward. "The depression created other issues in me—overeating, and the online purchases started, and I spent so much money," she shared when we reconnected months after our sessions working together. "[The online shopping] was a bind for me, and I really thought, I don't know how I could ever stop doing this. I also had an issue with clutter."

After tapping together in multiple sessions, in addition to being able to resume yoga and a normal, active life again, Tara was able to stop her online spending and clear the clutter in her home. These changes didn't feel difficult. They were just things she didn't want to do anymore. That often happens when we clear the underlying issues related to pain. Other limiting patterns, issues, and blocks in our lives fall away because we feel better about ourselves. As a result, we no longer want to self-sabotage or avoid what isn't working in our lives. Instead, we want to do the things that make us feel good. As we've seen, this process can also work in reverse. By first tapping through issues around relationships, finances, work, and other things, some people get the pain relief they've been hoping for.

It's another reminder that pain and pain relief aren't just about the presence or absence of pain. Becoming pain-free is about clearing the underlying emotions and beliefs, and it's also about looking at your overall life choices. Even if you've already gotten pain relief by this point, it's important to take an honest and thorough look at your life. Any areas of your life that are a constant source of stress need to be addressed. If they're not, your pain is more likely to return. And even if they're not related to the pain, we might as well live the most abundant, happy, and stress-free life possible!

With your journal and a pen or pencil in hand, begin to look at the different parts of your life—your relationships, work, finances, home, lifestyle (diet, exercise, schedule, home environment), and so on. Does your lifestyle support your health and wellness? Are your relationships adding to or taking away from your emotional, mental, and physical well-being? What about your job, how you spend your time, even where you live?

While we won't be able to address all of these issues individually here, it's important that you begin to notice what is and isn't working in your life. It's time to take an honest inventory of the parts of your life that need more attention, begin tapping on what's not working, and take action to make changes when and where necessary.

If it feels too overwhelming to look at your entire life all at once, begin tapping through the points while asking yourself the following questions: *What in my life is stressing me out? What do I worry about most often? What makes me anxious, angry, and/or afraid?* Make notes in your journal of everything you discover and commit to tapping through each issue, one by one.

Tuning In vs. Tuning Out

When we're talking about ways to take care of ourselves, it's important to differentiate between tuning *in* to what makes us feel good—the people, activities, and pursuits that "fill us up"—versus the things that allow us to tune *out*.

TV, the Internet, and digital devices are all amusing, sometimes necessary, distractions. They allow us to tune out, but they can't provide the level of fulfillment and engagement that hobbies and passions like making music, doing yoga, gardening, and others do. There's nothing wrong with using technology and enjoying the entertainment it can provide, but to practice real self-care, we often need to spend more time on the activities and people that "fill us up" rather than just steal our attention away from what's happening in the body and our lives.

The All-Knowing Knees: Your Body and Exercise

One specific area I encourage all my pain clients to look at is their relationship with their body and exercise. Once Kevin had tapped through and cleared the emotional charge from traumatic childhood memories, I knew it was time to address his relationship with his body. "Is there any hope for your body healing?" I asked. "That's not what the medical community tells me," he replied as he continued tapping through the points. "What do you think?" I asked. "I would like to think that there is," he answered.

Kevin had undergone hip-replacement surgery on both of his hips and been diagnosed with severe spinal stenosis. For years, he had suffered from chronic pain in his neck, feet, and right shoulder. The painkillers he took several times per day numbed the pain, but his body still felt broken. As he put it, "The worst of the pain is gone, but performance isn't really satisfactory." As a result, Kevin had become significantly overweight. The extra weight had further weakened his body and added to his pain.

"Can you find a sliver of hope?" I asked next. "Yes, in my knees. They're the one major joint that's never had any problems," he replied.

"Rock-solid knees," I offered.

"Yes, always served me well," he responded. I asked him to think of a name for his knees and to begin tapping through the points as we continued.

After several moments of silence, he offered, "The All-Knowing Knees."

To make it fun and add a visual component to the process, I asked his knees to call a meeting. "Hear, hear! The all-knowing knees, calling a meeting to order," I began. "Calling in the right shoulder. Can you see the right shoulder limping in?" I asked.

"Low crawling," Kevin noted.

"Okay, the right shoulder is low crawling into the meeting. Now calling in the neck!" I continued.

"The neck is limping in," he explained.

"What other parts of the body are called to this meeting?" I asked.

"My left foot. It has tendon issues. It's flopping in. My right foot, too; it's dragging," he said. I continued to ask him what other body parts needed to attend this meeting. "My eyes—they look kind of crossed. And my spine—it's all plugged up," he said.

"Picture them all in the meeting," I guided him. "See those knees that have hope, the knees that are hope. What do they say to this straggly bunch?" I asked.

"First of all, my knees have drill sergeant hats on," he said.

"Perfect! What do they say?" I asked.

"Look, you bunch of wimps, get with the program! Line up the way you're supposed to. Do your job!" he said.

"What else do they want to say?" I asked.

"Enjoy your work," he said, adding, "and when you're done, at ease."

By identifying with the strong part of his body—his knees—Kevin could begin to create a positive, empowering relationship with his body. Within just a few minutes, he was able to envision how he wanted his body to work. He wanted it to perform when it needed to and relax and enjoy the rest of the time.

"So you've got a bunch of cadets here that need a bit of work," I continued.

"Absolutely," Kevin replied, still tapping through the points.

"Just hold that image of your knees whipping them all into shape," I guided him.

"Get down and give me five," he continued. "Get in shape so you can do your job."

"You've got to exercise to get in shape, and it's going to be a little painful sometimes during the workout," I said, wanting to test the strength of his new relationship with his body and exercise.

"No pain, no gain," Kevin replied.

"How's the rest of the body responding to this?" I asked as we continued tapping.

"They're falling into formation," he replied.

"Beautiful," I responded, "and now they have a leader. Maybe that's what they needed all along."

"I'm sure it is," he said as he continued tapping through the points.

"Now [your body parts] have a vision for the future. They see those knees, and how well they work," I guided him. "Feel that strength in your body. Your spine is getting stronger; your neck and shoulders and feet are getting stronger. Can you feel that strength? Can you feel that confidence?" I asked.

"Absolutely, I can. It feels looser, more fluid . . . not as grinding, not as dry," he replied.

"Know that you can go back to that place at any time, with your knees leading the way. You can be strong again. You can be the man that you are. You can be the man you've always wanted to be. You can be strong *and* vulnerable, courageous *and* loving, passionate *and* peaceful," I added.

When we were done tapping, I asked Kevin how his body felt. The pain in his neck had gone from a 5 out of 10 to a 1 out of 10; his shoulder had gone from a 5 out of 10 down to a 0 out of 10. Just as important, he'd begun a new relationship with his body. His knees had become a source of strength. He could rely on them to lead the rest of his body forward. Together, they could rebuild physical strength and regain flexibility through regular exercise, which is critical to having and maintaining a healthy, strong, pain-free body.

Strengthening Your Body

Because pain limits movement, it almost universally leads to weakened muscles and, eventually, frail bones. As your physical body becomes weaker, you become more prone to pain and injury. For long-term pain relief, it's critical that you begin to incorporate regular physical exercise into your life. According to John

Sarno, M.D., author of *Healing Back Pain,* resuming regular exercise is one of the best things you can do to relieve pain:

> One must do this not simply for the sake of becoming a normal human being again (though that is a good enough reason physically and psychologically by itself) but to liberate oneself from the fear of physical activity, which is often more effective than pain in keeping one's mind focused on the body . . . Losing one's fear and resuming normal physical activity is possibly the most important part of the therapeutic process.

For many people, the idea of more pain prevents them from exercising, and it's that fear of more pain, rather than the physical activity itself, that's the biggest barrier to resuming regular physical activity. Because the fear of exercise increasing pain is often intense enough to negatively impact the body, Sarno advises resuming exercise only once you believe that exercise will help alleviate your pain:

> Never do this or that, do it this way, we're told; be careful, you'll hurt yourself; your spine is out of line; the discs are degenerated and the spinal bones are rubbing together; one of your legs is shorter than the other; people weren't meant to walk upright; you've got flat feet; don't swim the crawl or the breast stroke; don't arch your back; never sleep on your stomach; always bend your knees when you bend at the waist or come back up; don't lift; don't do sit-ups, do crunches; and on and on.
>
> All of these admonitions and prohibitions, enhanced by poor medical advice, keep your attention riveted on your body, which is your brain's intention.
>
> The path to resumption of full physical activity, without fear, may be slow and uneven. Don't worry if you begin to exercise too soon and experience some pain. You cannot hurt yourself; TMS [a disease in which chronic pain results from repressed emotions like anger and sadness] is a benign process. Continuing pain with activity means the brain is still in the process of changing its programming. You must bide your time, try and try again, and stay secure in the knowledge that you will prevail in the end. This has proven to be the case for thousands of patients.
>
> On the other hand, don't start the physical program too soon—not because of potential physical harm, but because the brain may still be programmed in the TMS mode. I recommend waiting a few weeks after

you accept the TMS diagnosis so the pain can diminish, confidence can be strengthened, and the brain will have had time to be reprogrammed.

In making the case for resuming physical exercise, Sarno adds:

> It should be noted, parenthetically, that the advice to resume normal physical activity, including the most vigorous, has been given to a very large number of patients over the past seventeen years. I cannot recall one person who has subsequently said that this advice caused him or her to have further back trouble.

While Sarno's approach seems radical to some, outside research confirms his findings. In one study published by *BMJ*, formerly known as the *British Medical Journal*, 187 patients between the ages of 18 and 60 who had had low back pain were monitored over a 12-month period. They were randomly divided into two groups. Only the intervention group was led through a program that included physical exercise, while the nonintervention group received only standard primary care treatment for back pain. After six weeks, the intervention group, which was exercising regularly, showed modest improvement over the nonintervention group. After six months, the intervention group showed significant improvement over the nonexercisers. At the one-year mark, the intervention group was still exercising and showed significant pain relief. The regular exercisers also had less need for medical intervention to manage their back pain and took significantly fewer days off of work.

Dr. James Rainville, chief of physical medicine and rehabilitation at New England Baptist Hospital in Boston, Massachusetts, has also demonstrated the power of exercise in alleviating pain. For his patients with moderate to severe back pain, he runs a program known as the "back pain boot camp," which was featured on National Public Radio (NPR) because of its success rates, which are higher than those of back surgery and painkillers.

Dr. Rainville's "boot camp" is a rigorous six-week exercise program that's focused on building strength and flexibility throughout the body, especially the back. Throughout the entire program, patients walk, run, lift weights, do aerobics, and more. By the end of the program, many experience significant, if not total, pain relief. During the six-week period, patients also regain enough strength and mobility to resume normal, active lives. Many also experience higher energy levels, better sleep, and other benefits, like weight loss and improved moods.

Exercise and the Fear of Reinjury

Since 2003, my friend Stacey Vornbrock, M.S., L.P.C., has worked with hundreds of elite and amateur athletes, using tapping to improve performance and also overcome a common fear, which is the fear of reinjury. Her Injury Recovery Program covers many aspects of an injury, including two of the most important ones, which are the fear of reinjury and the memory of protection.

Many of her clients have experienced chronic pain, as well as multiple injuries to multiple parts of the body. Here's what she shared with me about the fear of reinjury:

When you are injured, multiple chemicals are released on the cellular level, including all the emotions (which are chemicals), and they are stored in the cell receptors around the injured area. Immediately your body takes on a fear of reinjury and develops a memory of protection around the injured area, and you begin to move in a way to protect the part of your body that was injured. You are now open to additional injuries because you are not moving, running, walking, making plays, and so on, in your normal way.

The most important thing to understand is that the fear of reinjury and the memory of protection remain in place forever, unless they are released on the cellular level. The more injuries you have, the more your body experiences fear and tightness. Your body adapts to performing with this fear, but you will not be able to perform at your true potential as long as the fear of reinjury and memory of protection remain in the cells.

Athletes are very aware of this fear of reinjury and holding back physically after an injury, but they keep trying to mentally overcome this. Unfortunately, it isn't possible for them to think their way out of this, but with tapping this can easily be released from the body. My athletes return to their preinjury level of performance after we tap.

Here's an example of how the fear of reinjury affected one of my athletes:

I worked with an 18-year-old man who was a gymnast at the top of his division in USA Gymnastics. He was concerned with his inconsistency in some of his routines, specifically pommel, high bar, and floor. Of course these three routines were the routines where he had fallen the most and been injured.

Here's a list of his injuries: both ankles sprained at least ten times; giant bruise on his foot after his foot hit the bar on his dismount; multiple falls off the pommel; left wrist sprain; injured his back and ankle when he landed short on a vault dismount (he could feel his spine crack); twisted his knee on a landing on his floor routine.

As a result of these injuries, every time he had to land a routine, he was aware of his body tensing up and holding back during his dismount. Of course, this opened his body up to further injuries and he wasn't performing at the level he knew he was capable of. Imagine the sheer willpower and energy it took to overcome his fear of falling and getting hurt every time he landed during practices and performances. Rather than just emptying his mind and letting his body perform the routine, he was distracted with the anticipation of the landing.

We tapped while focusing on releasing the fear of reinjury and the memory of protection for each injury. We also tapped to release his fear with each apparatus and all landings from each apparatus. Then we tapped to put his body in harmony with each apparatus to create a harmonic resonance that allowed his body to naturally be in tune and at ease with each apparatus.

His goal was to place in the top 50 at Nationals the year we worked together. He ended up placing in the top 5 in the overall competition, completely exceeding the goal he'd set for himself!

Creating a New Relationship with Exercise

While much of the research on the benefits of exercise in alleviating chronic pain has been focused on back pain, it's important to understand that regular exercise is central to long-lasting pain relief throughout the body. It's also crucial to overall health and wellness. The key is to address how you feel exercise will impact your body and your pain.

To begin creating a positive relationship with exercise, let's do some tapping now on overcoming fears that exercise will create more pain.

When you think about exercising potentially causing you pain, how do you feel? Give your emotions a number of intensity on a scale of 0 to 10. Also give your pain its own number. Write both of these down in your journal. Now start tapping:

Karate Chop: Even though I am convinced that exercise is painful for me, I accept that's how I feel right now.

Karate Chop: Even though I'm sure it will be painful for me to exercise, because it was in the past, I accept myself even with these fears.

Karate Chop: Even though exercise has been painful for me before and I'm sure it will be again, I'm open to being surprised with a different outcome.

Eyebrow: I can't exercise because it's painful . . .

Side of Eye: I know my body will rebel if I exercise.

Under Eye: I've paid the price before for exercise . . .

Under Nose: I'm sure that my body will be mad at me.

Chin: It will get stiff and sore . . .

Collarbone: It's just not worth it.

Under Arm: Exercise is hard!

Top of Head: I don't have the time to exercise.

Eyebrow: I'm scared to move my body . . .

Side of Eye: I'm not sure I can trust my body to be strong.

Under Eye: My body has let me down before . . .

Under Nose: And I don't know how to trust it again.

Chin: Perhaps I could be easy with my body . . .

Collarbone: Allowing my body to grow stronger . . .

Under Arm: Take small steps . . .

Top of Head: But still, I'm scared to move my body.

Check in with yourself and notice how you're feeling about exercise now. Give it a number on a scale of 0 to 10. Keep tapping on the "negative" until the intensity is a 5 or lower and then switch to some positive rounds. Also notice if your pain has shifted. Remember, these scripts are just here for guidance and to get you started. Feel free to use your own language, speak your own truth, and so forth.

Positive Round

Eyebrow: What if I were a mover . . .

Side of Eye: I could find enjoyment in moving . . .

Under Eye: I love knowing it can be simple!

Under Nose: I love knowing there are so many ways for me to be a mover!

Chin: When I move I am taking part in life . . .

Collarbone: I'm engaging my body in a playful way . . .

Under Arm: I could be surprised to find that my body wants to move!

Top of Head: I could be surprised that my body enjoys moving.

Take a deep breath and think again about exercising. How do you feel about it now? Give it a number on a scale of 0 to 10. Keep tapping until your emotional intensity is a 3 or lower—even if it takes 20 minutes of tapping. Also check in on your pain and notice any shifts you may have experienced.

Moving Toward a New Future

As you work through what isn't working in your life and incorporate new ways of thinking, being, and living that support pain relief, your self-love and self-acceptance will naturally expand. The next step is to create a bigger vision for your life, a vision that goes beyond pain relief.

Audio Bonus: To do more tapping on creating a new relationship with your body, join me in a free audio tapping meditation here: thetappingsolution .com/painbookresources.

CHAPTER 10

CREATING A HEALTHY, ABUNDANT, PAIN-FREE VISION FOR YOUR FUTURE

When you envision your future, what do you see? Can you imagine yourself living a healthy, pain-free, and abundant life? Can you see yourself, your body, and your life getting better every day?

Ultimately, this process has to be about more than pain relief. It needs to be about moving forward in a new way, leaving old patterns behind, and investing in a healthy, abundant, and, yes, pain-free vision for your future. So let's get started!

Doing the Little Things You Used to Love

You can begin creating a new vision for your life by doing the little things you loved to do before you had pain. For Sarah, that meant running a few steps with her dog, Tiger. "This morning," she shared, "I was out with Tiger, and he was in such a silly mood, and I found myself running down the sidewalk with him, just caught up in the moment. And then I thought, *Oh no, my hip is really going to pay me back for that,* because usually when I let myself run, my hip will throb for hours, or even a day or two. But this time, after doing all that tapping, there was nothing, no pain. So I thought, *Hmm, let's try that again.* So Tiger and I continued to be silly and run down the sidewalk, and I'm absolutely fine!"

These small daily acts that bring you pleasure are more important than you realize. They change your physiology and prompt your body to release good hormones and chemicals that contribute to pain relief. It's a powerful place of healing and wellness that can do wonders for you and your body. Just running those few steps with her dog transformed Sarah's entire day and gave her a sense of hope that opened up new possibilities for her future. And even though she expected the pain to return, because she had tapped, it never did.

What simple daily pleasures have fallen out of your life because of your pain? Get your journal now and make a list of simple, everyday acts that would make you feel good. Whether it's a walk in nature, a few minutes spent playing with your animals and/or children, playing an instrument, calling a friend who makes you laugh, or something else, write them all down now.

If the thought of doing something that falls outside your ordinary routine scares you, do some tapping on it now. Begin by rating the intensity of your emotions on a scale of 0 to 10. Give your pain a separate number, write both numbers in your journal, and then start tapping:

Karate Chop: Even though I have this anxiety about getting back out there again, I accept myself and these feelings.

Karate Chop: Even though up till now my pain has kept me from taking any risks or trying something new, I still accept myself and I choose to know that I'm okay.

Karate Chop: Even though I have these fears and apprehensions about trying new things, I'm willing to give it a try.

Eyebrow: This anxiety about putting myself out there . . .

Side of Eye: What if I can't handle it . . .

Under Eye: What if it's overwhelming . . .

Under Nose: People will expect so much from me . . .

Chin: How will I protect myself . . .

Collarbone: What if my pain comes back . . .

Under Arm: What if I overdo it . . .

Top of Head: There is so much pressure to try something new when I no longer have this pain.

Eyebrow: It's overwhelming . . .

Side of Eye: It's too much.

Under Eye: I can't do it.

Under Nose: There are too many risks out there!

Chin: I won't be able to handle it all.

Collarbone: And yet I choose to remember . . .

Under Arm: That I've been growing and learning.

Top of Head: It feels overwhelming, but I've got new skills and resources.

Check in with yourself and notice how you're feeling emotionally. Give your emotions a number on a scale of 0 to 10. Keep tapping on the "negative" until the intensity is a 5 or lower, and then switch to some positive rounds. Also check in to see if your pain has shifted. Remember, these scripts are just here for guidance and to get you started. Feel free to use your own language, speak your own truth, and so forth.

Positive Round

Eyebrow: I can tap when I'm overwhelmed . . .

Side of Eye: I have learned to set boundaries.

Under Eye: I remember that I can ask for what I need.

Under Nose: I remember that I can say no when I need to.

Chin: I remember that I'm learning to listen to my body . . .

Collarbone: To respect and honor my needs . . .

Under Arm: I am ready to be part of life again!

Top of Head: I trust the wisdom in me now.

When you're ready, rate the intensity of your emotions on a scale of 0 to 10. Also notice any shifts in your pain. Once the intensity of your emotions is a 3 or lower, go do one activity on your list, even if it's only for a few minutes. Take that time to make your own enjoyment a priority. Remember, sometimes the best thing you can do is to stop focusing on the pain and start focusing on the things that make you feel good. Over time your brain will get the message that your happiness is more important than your pain.

* *

Small daily acts that bring you pleasure are more important than you realize. They change your physiology and prompt your body to release good hormones and chemicals that contribute to pain relief. It's a powerful place of healing and wellness that can do wonders for you and your body.

* *

Expanding on the Positive

As you move toward wellness and pleasure, and away from pain and limitation, it's important to make a conscious effort to notice and surround yourself with as much positive input as possible. Do your tapping and enjoy the stress relief and relaxation it provides. Spend more time with people who love and support you. Do activities you enjoy. Eat healthy food that nourishes your body and gives you energy. Spend more time moving your body. As often as possible, focus on all the things you can do and think about that make you feel good.

In his number-one international bestseller, *The Science of Happiness*, author Stefan Klein, Ph.D., explains why it's important to make a conscious effort to focus on the positive:

> Someone who has learned to contain his dark moods and to fortify his sunny ones is also taking care of his body. Positive feelings counteract stress and its consequences for health. They even stimulate the immune system.

Tapping is an especially powerful way to experience more positive feelings because it allows you to quiet your amygdala, the primitive part of the brain programmed for survival (this is where the negativity bias we learned about earlier kicks into high gear, always scanning for threats) as you encode positive experiences into your brain.

As Klein shares, training your brain to focus on the positive supports you in two important ways:

Happiness can be both one of life's goals, and the means to a better life. Negative moods limit people, whereas positive feelings expand options. Happiness brings vitality.

He later adds:

Feelings of happiness aren't a coincidence but the consequence of right thought and actions—a concept with which modern neuroscience, ancient philosophy, and Buddhism (which believes in a strict principle of cause and effect) all agree.

The good news is, Klein explains, we can train our brains to experience more happiness:

Two things are certain. First, our sense of happiness depends much more on the ways in which the brain perceives than on external circumstances; and second, occasional efforts aren't sufficient to change our ways of perceiving. If the brain is to be rewired, repetition and habit are indispensable. And they, in turn, depend on a willingness to make an effort.

People are willing to go to great lengths when it concerns status, career, or their children's development. But when it concerns happiness in everyday life, they can be oddly stingy with their energy. And yet, the way to happiness is quite straightforward: "The actual secrets of the path to happiness are determination, effort and time," explains the Dalai Lama.

To this, science can only assent.

Rather than letting positive thoughts and experiences fade away, do some tapping on them throughout your day. Whenever your pain goes down, tap on how good your body feels. Go stand in the sunshine and tap while letting yourself feel how good that light and warmth feels on your skin. Stop to notice a pretty flower, smell it, and tap while you feel that appreciation and enjoyment.

These moments may feel weird, even forced, at first. That's normal—after all, you're actively working against your brain's ingrained negativity bias. Remember, your goal here isn't to pretend that everything's great when it isn't. By tapping in the positive in addition to tapping to clear the negative, you're expanding your ability to appreciate and feel the positive. In *Hardwiring Happiness,* Hanson explains it this way:

> When you tilt toward the good, you're not denying or resisting the bad. You're simply acknowledging, enjoying, and using the good. You're aware of the whole truth, *all* the tiles of the mosaic of life, not only the negative ones. You recognize the good in yourself, in others, in the world, and in the future we can make together. And when you choose to, you take it in.

So if you have pain, or if you just had a fight with a loved one, tap on what's actually true. Tap on the anger and frustration you feel. Once you've cleared that, also take the time to appreciate how much calmer you feel after tapping, as well as any other positive thoughts or emotions that come to you. Again, by tapping on the positive as well as the negative, you're creating more balance in your brain. You're giving the positive stuff a chance to stick.

Appreciating What *Is* Working in Your Body

As we discussed before, appreciating what does work in your body is a powerful act—and it goes exactly along with your work to combat the negativity bias. So start noticing the parts of your body that are healthy and that do feel good. Make a list of each one and express your gratitude toward every one of them as you tap through the points.

I know this seems ironic, but it's also important to notice the negative influences that surround you. Many of them are so ingrained in our culture that we forget to notice. Think about it. When you turn on the television, open your e-mail, or flip through a magazine, you rarely see ads about tapping and meditation. Instead, you see ads for the insurance you should have and the cars, homes, beer, food, and clothes you should buy. Unfortunately, a lot of the media we're exposed to hundreds of times a day use fear and negativity as tools to convince you to spend more money on the products and services they're selling. The underlying message is that you're in danger, or that you and your life are not good enough.

To break out of the patterns that led to your being in chronic pain, it's a good idea to distance yourself from these negative influences. You need to make an effort every day to let more positive than negative information into your brain, your life, your home, and your relationships. Do what you need to do to let the positive outweigh the negative.

. . . .

Rather than letting positive thoughts and experiences fade away, do some tapping on them throughout your day. Whenever your pain goes down, tap on how good your body feels. Go stand in the sunshine and tap while letting yourself feel how good that light and warmth feels on your skin. Stop to notice a pretty flower, smell it, and tap while you feel that appreciation and enjoyment.

. . . .

I do this for myself every day. In addition to the time I spend tapping, I pack my iPod with audio teachings from inspirational leaders I admire. I listen to them over and over again to instill positive energy and messages into my brain and body. There are audios in there I've probably listened to 500 times, and I'll probably listen to them another 500 times. They keep me feeling positive and functioning at a higher level.

Keep in mind, there is no one "right" way to bring more positive influences into your life. And this process of emphasizing positive inputs over negative ones isn't necessarily about making sudden or drastic changes in your life.

To the greatest degree possible, try to surround yourself with people, places, activities, and other input that make you feel good. Also notice what you're thinking about and how you're feeling. Tap through negative emotions and thoughts as often as you can so that you can spend more time feeling good and thinking positive thoughts.

What to Do Less Of:

- Watching television
- Reading and watching the news
- Gossiping
- Eating junk food, processed food, sugar
- Taking mind-altering substances
- Smoking
- Always noticing what you don't like
- Never noticing what you do enjoy
- Remaining physically inactive
- Spending time with negative people

What to Do More Of:

- Tapping
- Doing things that make you feel good
- Taking part in physical activity
- Eating fresh, healthy food that nourishes and energizes you
- Noticing what in your body is working
- Appreciating moments when you feel good
- Spending time around people who love and support you
- Noticing what you love about people
- Reading books that inspire you
- Listening to inspiring audios
- Attending events that inspire you
- Pursuing personal hobbies and passions

Have Patience with Yourself—It Takes Time

Throughout this book, I've said that using tapping to achieve total pain relief is a process, an ongoing journey. If you haven't yet gotten the pain relief you're seeking, you may be feeling even more impatient, more anxious and frustrated than ever. (Tap on it!)

Wherever you are in your journey, it's important to remember that it took 10, 20, 40, even 60 or more years to create the emotional, mental, and physiological patterns that got you to a place of chronic pain. Those patterns have become deeply ingrained in your brain, your body, your relationships, and your life. Most people can't undo those patterns by reading this book once or by tapping occasionally. This is a process, and you need to give it time. If that means reading and rereading this book and tapping through it five or ten times, do it!

As we've seen, the issues behind the pain are multilayered, and this is a process of peeling the onion, one layer at a time. If you haven't yet gotten pain relief, or if your pain returns because you stop tapping and return to your old patterns of not taking care of yourself, it may feel easier to give up on this process than to dive in even deeper with your tapping. But your unconscious mind *wants* you to give up on pain relief. It will convince you that tapping doesn't apply to you or your condition; that you don't have time or energy to make changes in your life; that you don't have the money/time/freedom/etc. to live the life you really want. Tap on all of it!

• •

Remember that it took 10, 20, 40, even 60 or more years to create the emotional, mental, and physiological patterns that got you to a place of chronic pain. Those patterns have become deeply ingrained in your brain, your body, your relationships, and your life. Most people can't undo those patterns by reading this book once or by tapping occasionally. This is a process, and you need to give it time.

• •

Remembering to Tap Daily

Incorporating tapping into your daily life takes practice, too! Here are a few ways of reminding yourself:

- Put a Post-It note that says "Tap Today!" on your bathroom mirror.

- Put a note on your bedside table.

- Put a daily reminder on your digital calendar.

Ultimately it's your responsibility to continue this process, to stay focused on pain relief, health, and wellness, as well as tapping, even on the days when you want to give up. Your job is to keep moving forward. On days when you're not feeling your best, you'll discover a million reasons, which are all valid, for abandoning this journey. It's up to you to stay committed to getting the pain relief you're seeking and then to creating the life you want to live.

That's why it's so important to create a bigger vision for yourself and your future. If the end result of this process is limited to being pain-free, as exciting as that is, it's not enough to break the old patterns that led to chronic pain in the first place. Unless and until you expand on your vision for what's possible for you, you can't expect to fully escape the patterns that contributed to your chronic pain.

One client I'd been working with for a few months shared that her ongoing process was productive but inconsistent. "Things are definitely shifting, so that's good," she began. As she continued to tap on her own nearly every day, her pain had been moving to new places in her body, which had never happened before tapping. She'd also pinpointed the root emotional cause of her pain, but she was continuing to discover new layers, like anger at herself for being overweight and letting her career go.

Some days she still struggled with the process. "There's still a part of me that just wants to be 90, and to look back and say, 'It's done—I did what I had to do in this life,'" she explained, "and I feel guilty about that." After spending more than two decades taking care of a demanding family while also coping with financial limitations, she felt exhausted and didn't know how to take care of herself. Obstacles kept appearing in her life, and it felt like too much at times.

"But," she continued, "I'm really determined to get better, so I'm not giving up. I'm tapping, and I'm going to get this out of my body one way or another."

In spite of her ups and downs, her good and bad days, she was refusing to give up. She was determined to overcome and move beyond the challenges she was facing in her circumstances, emotions, body, and finances. That's what this journey, and any important journey, ultimately requires.

Oprah is an amazing example of someone who has overcome incredible odds to create the life of her dreams. Born to an unwed teenage mother, starting at the age of nine she was abused by multiple men, including her own relatives. After trying to run away, she was sent to a juvenile detention home but was turned away because they didn't have any available beds. By the age of 14, she was on her own and, soon after, gave birth to a baby who died in infancy. And those details are only a few of the obstacles Oprah has faced and overcome!

Louise Hay's story is similarly inspiring. She grew up poor and was abused as a teenager. After being diagnosed with cancer, she used the methods that she would later publish in her best-selling book *You Can Heal Your Life* to become cancer-free within six months. She would then go on to found Hay House—my publisher and one of the leaders in the self-help and personal development industry—at the age of 58.

When we read stories like that, we don't assume we're talking about people who have helped to heal millions of people around the world. Both Oprah and Louise—and many, many others—have been able to create the life and success they have by persevering through incredibly challenging circumstances.

Needless to say, I'm not suggesting that you need to change the world, start an industry, or become a billionaire. I am telling you that you may need a similar level of resolve and commitment to get out of your old patterns and create new ones that contribute to pain relief, health, and wellness, as well as abundance, love, and anything else you want in your life.

This is a journey, and if you want to live a healthy, pain-free, and abundant life, you're going to have to tap on days when you don't feel like it. You're going to need to strengthen your body through exercise even though it feels uncomfortable. You're going to need to take care of your body by eating fresh, nourishing food, and you may also need to make changes in your relationships, your work, and other parts of your life you'd rather not face.

What Does Your Future Look Like?

One important way to move yourself forward is by noticing the story you tell yourself about your future. Now that you've read and hopefully tapped through this book, can you envision a pain-free future for yourself? Can you imagine achieving other goals? Reaching a new level of abundance? Being in a loving, committed relationship? Being physically active and healthy? Losing weight or starting the business you've always dreamed of owning? Whatever it is you want for yourself and in your life, can you really see that being *your* life?

Oprah tells a great story about growing up with her grandmother, who called her over as a young girl to teach her how to churn the butter. Understandably, her grandmother assumed that Oprah, too, would have to churn her own butter someday. Oprah remembers, even as a young child, thinking something like, *Oh, no, Grandma, I won't need to churn my own butter.* Even at that young age, she had a larger vision for her future. That vision helped her move toward her dreams in spite of the incredible challenges she faced over many years.

ASK YOURSELF: After reading and tapping through the pain-relief process in this book, what story are you telling yourself? Are you telling yourself that every time you tap you're moving toward a pain-free, healthy, and abundant future? Or are you telling yourself that your pain will never go away or that it will eventually return?

These stories that live inside us are powerful. They're the difference between tapping or not tapping, taking better care of ourselves or not, and paying more attention to what is and isn't working in our lives. Almost anything, including permanent pain relief, is possible if you're willing to believe in it, because that belief will give you the energy and motivation to continue tapping, to attend events that inspire you, to read inspirational books, or do whatever else it is that makes you feel alive and inspired to move beyond any limitations you may be facing.

Let's do some tapping now on moving beyond old stories of what is and isn't possible for you and creating a larger vision for your future.

When you think about moving beyond your old story and creating a pain-free, healthy, and abundant future, how possible does it seem? Give it a number on a scale of 0 to 10, rate your pain separately, write both in your journal, and then start tapping:

Karate Chop: Even though I've had this old story for so long, and it's been a part of who I am, I choose to remember that I am more than this old story.

Karate Chop: Even though a part of me will miss this old story, the one about the pain and limitations, I know there is a part of me that is ready to move on.

Karate Chop: Even though I'm not sure who I will be with another story, I accept all of me, without this old story.

Eyebrow: I've been carrying around this old story for as long as I can remember . . .

Side of Eye: I thought I was this story.

Under Eye: It's been a sad story . . .

Under Nose: There has been a lot of drama in it . . .

Chin: Thank goodness the story isn't over yet!

Collarbone: I get to write the ending to that story.

Under Arm: I can make this an amazing story . . .

Top of Head: I can make it a story about healing . . .

Eyebrow: And about discovery . . .

Side of Eye: About new beginnings . . .

Under Eye: And possibilities.

Under Nose: I get to be the star of this new story!

Chin: And even though the first few chapters were rough . . .

Collarbone: This can be an amazing story now.

Under Arm: My new story is full of grace . . .

Top of Head: My new story is full of wonder.

Eyebrow: My new story is being written right now.

Side of Eye: I am the star!

Under Eye: I am the producer.

Under Nose: I am the director.

Chin: I am the hero or heroine!

Collarbone: I choose a story that captures the best parts of me.

Under Arm: I am the story I choose to write.

Top of Head: I write a beautiful story now.

Take a deep breath and check in with yourself. How possible does your new story feel now? How relevant does your old story feel now? Give it a number on a scale of 0 to 10. Keep tapping until your old story feels true at a 3 or lower—even if it takes 20 minutes of tapping. Also take note of any shifts in your pain.

Get Support!

None of us can accomplish great things entirely on our own. We all need support. When I was making my documentary and then building my business, I made a point of surrounding myself with mentors and friends who wanted to see me succeed, people who wanted to support me. I still do, and I could never have gotten to where I am without that support.

Getting support is just as critical for you in this journey toward a pain-free, healthy, and abundant future. Make a point of seeking out people who can give you that support. So many of the people who attended my pain-relief events comment on how healing it was to be with other people who were committed to getting pain relief and healing themselves and their lives. After events, some of them connected on Facebook and continued to interact online and support each other in moving forward. I really can't stress enough the importance of getting this kind of positive support!

Especially if you're the kind of person who's always been self-sufficient, always feeling like you have to do things by yourself, it's time to step back, notice that belief, and tap on it. Acknowledge that your "I have to do it all alone" belief may be one of the patterns that is contributing to your chronic pain. Then find people who are also seeking out health and wellness and who want to connect. Help each other move forward, one step at a time. You'll be amazed by what becomes possible when you have even one person who's there to support you.

Everything's Shifting . . . and It's Effortless!

Bobbie got in touch with me almost exactly four months after I'd worked with her onstage, tapping with the audience through her memory of her father telling her at her fifth birthday party that he wished she'd never been born. I was thrilled to hear about the changes that had taken place in her and her life since that day.

"First and foremost," she began, "my marriage has gotten so much better. Before tapping with you on that memory of my dad, I was distancing myself from my husband. I was disconnecting because I didn't feel supported or understood. Since that day, though, there's been a gradual shift of where my attention is. I've been paying more attention to the things I love about him. Just a few weeks ago, at our anniversary dinner, he mentioned that he'd noticed how I'd been appreciating him more, and I was like, 'Yeah, I have,' and it opened up this amazing conversation. The intimacy and everything between us has improved by leaps and bounds. I actually *want* to connect with him now, whereas before I was avoiding it like the plague . . . before tapping through those memories of my dad, I think my husband had gotten lumped in with my dad. He was doing what my dad said a man never would. He was loving and accepting me as I was, and that made my dad wrong."

Just as the pain isn't just about the pain, the issues behind the pain, like Bobbie's memories of her dad, don't just contribute to pain. They also hold us back in our relationships and throughout our lives. Once the issues behind the pain are cleared, it's not just the pain that goes away. It's all the old beliefs and repressed emotions that have been holding us back. With those gone, we're free to step into the life we've always dreamed of living.

"Having all those people say that my dad was wrong," she continued, "changed everything, even my relationship with my boys." Before she tapped through her dad's memory that day, she explained, her relationship with her youngest son had always been strained. Since tapping, however, their relationship has completely changed. She's been able to appreciate their differences. "It's not a battle anymore. It's just comfortable."

Talking to Bobbie, I was struck by how energized and excited she sounded. It was a huge difference! We talked for several minutes about her life in general before we even discussed how she was feeling physically. When we did, she said, "My left knee pain has not come back." This was after 25 years of relentless knee pain that had controlled her life. Then she added, "The only pain I've been experiencing in my body is from all the exercise I'm doing!" In addition to other forms of regular exercise, she had returned to her favorite winter sport, cross-country skiing, which she hadn't done for more than 20 years.

I was blown away by how much had transformed in Bobbie's life in such a short period of time. "Everything's shifting, and it's effortless," she explained. "I'm not having to fight for it." Since the pain-relief event, she'd also lost 25 pounds, stopped eating sugar, and barely watched television anymore. As a massage therapist who was in the process of getting certified as an EFT practitioner, Bobbie explained that she used to "veg out" in front of the TV between clients. Now, she explained, "If I have free time, I'm reading; sitting and vegging out between clients just isn't my primary thing anymore."

With all this new energy and possibility surrounding her, she's ready to step up in her career as well. "There are all these changes that keep adding up . . . It's organic. Just the other day," she shared, "I said to God, all right, God, I am ready for whatever it is I'm supposed to be doing . . . I've hidden under a rock for long enough, and I've cleared enough stuff that I'm finally ready to move forward. Bring me the people, circumstances, and opportunities I need for me to be doing what I am meant to be doing in this life."

Soon afterward, a client asked her to use his space to teach an EFT class. "I was like, absolutely! I just want to spread [EFT] as far and wide as I can," she explained. In the next few years, she sees herself teaching classes and working with clients, not just through massage but also with tapping.

Since this journey is different for everyone, I'm always curious about what makes the difference for people. When I asked Bobbie what had made the real difference for her, she replied, "I see it like a forest, and the biggest tree in the forest was my dad and what he'd said to me at that birthday party. It's like dominoes, and with that biggest tree down, the other trees are coming down effortlessly." As far as her knee pain was concerned, she added, "My dad was anchored to that knee, and when I let him go in love that day while tapping with the audience, it was like the chain just fell away."

Creating Your Vision

What does your dream life look like? All you need to do is begin to create it, knowing that you can continue to add to it as your vision expands.

Get your journal and take a look at the list you made earlier of simple everyday activities that bring you pleasure. Begin tapping through the points as you read through the list. Try to imagine how great each item on your list would make you feel. Dwell on all the enjoyment and positive feelings you'd experience.

Next, as you continue tapping through the points, begin asking yourself, *What else would I do or change if I could live my dream life?*

As ideas come to you, write them down. If nothing comes to you, you can also just write out in your journal what your perfect day would look like and expand on that over time.

As part of your ongoing tapping practice, begin to dwell on these visions of your dream life—your pain-free, healthy, and abundant life. As you tap while imagining it, let yourself feel how amazing you'll feel living this life. Try to do this positive tapping on your dreams on a daily basis, or as often as you can, in addition to tapping through any stress and negative emotions you experience. By tapping in this positive energy, you will increase your physical well-being and also build positive momentum for living this life you desire.

• •

As part of your ongoing tapping practice, begin to dwell on these visions of your dream life—your pain-free, healthy, and abundant life. As you tap while imagining it, let yourself feel how amazing you'll feel living this life.

• •

The Possibilities Are Endless

I always get excited when I get to work with someone who has chronic pain, whether it's on my weekly radio show or at a live event, because I know, without a doubt, that this process works. Over and over again, I've seen people with chronic pain and harsh, unforgiving diagnoses get lasting pain relief and heal the inner and outer wounds that have been controlling their lives.

The journey I've laid out in this book is different for everyone, and your journey can be whatever you want it to be. If you follow this process, and return to it whenever you need it, I know for sure that you will gain valuable insights into yourself, your emotions, and your pain. Be sure to celebrate every new insight, every shift, and every time you feel better. Use those moments as motivation to do more tapping and take better care of yourself. If you keep moving forward every day, 3, 6, and 12 months from now you'll be amazed by how different your body and your life feel.

I want to take a moment to acknowledge you and your courage, commitment, and burning desire to heal your body, to explore alternative, outside-the-box ways of finding pain relief and transforming your life. It takes a special kind of person to make this sort of commitment, and the fact that you've read this book, that you've made it to the end, that you're doing the tapping and healing your body and life, is incredible.

So thank you. Thank you for your commitment to yourself, to a better world, to healing. I would love to hear your success stories with tapping, so please share them with me at Nick@TheTappingSolution.com.

As I sign all my e-mails . . .

Until next time . . .
Take Care and Keep Tapping!

Audio Bonus: To do more tapping on creating a vibrant, pain-free vision of your future, join me in a free audio tapping meditation here: thetappingsolution .com/painbookresources.

THE STORY OF THE TAPPING SOLUTION FOUNDATION

As a result of this tapping work I've had the great fortune of doing, I've been able to share tapping with those who need it most, when they need it most—those who suffer from chronic pain and many others. That has never been truer than it is with the work I've been able to do through The Tapping Solution Foundation. It's an organization I never planned on founding, but one that has helped an enormous number of people in their darkest hours, and it has, in turn, enriched my life tremendously. I wanted to share the story of how the foundation came to be. Perhaps this story will inspire you to move your life forward in new ways by showing you what can become possible when you contribute your unique talents to people who really need them.

The Beginning of The Tapping Solution Foundation

"I don't know if you know this, but I live in Newtown." They were the first words out of my mouth when Dr. Lori Leyden, a psychologist and EFT practitioner, picked up the phone on December 15, 2012. The day before, 20 students and six adults had been shot and killed at Sandy Hook Elementary in my hometown.

Since hearing the news, I had been calling everyone I could think of to brainstorm what we could do to help the community.

After much discussion about the situation and what was possible, Lori and I laid out a plan. We would follow the same community-based model that Lori had been employing for several years in Rwanda through her nonprofit, Create Global Healing. That country, of course, was still healing from the enormous trauma caused by the 100-day-long genocide that led to the murder of 20 percent of the country's population in 1994. In addition to suffering deep emotional scars from all they had seen and experienced, like most PTSD sufferers, many Rwandans had also suffered from years of chronic pain. Lori and her team had transformed thousands of lives there: entire communities that had learned tapping had gotten the lasting pain relief, as well as the deep emotional healing, they needed to move forward and rebuild their country.

As Lori and I spoke on the phone that day, we decided to bring that same heart-centered approach to Newtown and create a community of EFT practitioners who could work with us and with the town to heal the community over time. We would come in quietly and begin by simply listening to the needs of the community and see how we could best serve. We wanted to give people in the community the chance to experience tapping, rather than force it on them.

Less than 72 hours later, Lori, who lives in Santa Barbara, California, was walking around Newtown with me, observing the evening funerals and wakes that were taking place throughout the town. As we walked, she talked about a heart-centered approach to trauma healing. "This is a new model for trauma healing, and we'll have to see if people here are open to it," she commented at one point.

A few minutes later, we both noticed a sign posted in a store window that read, "We are Sandy Hook. We choose love." We looked right at each other with tears in our eyes. There was a tremendous amount of work to be done, but we knew right then that we were in the right place.

During those early days in Newtown, we started just responding to calls that were coming in to The Tapping Solution, some from people volunteering their time, others from people seeking support. In the weeks that followed, as we worked with countless community members, we also began a rigorous training program for a group of 24 volunteer EFT practitioners. Our goal was to prepare them to work with trauma victims, which can take a toll on practitioners if they're not specifically trained for that kind of work.

Since that training, as a result of that group's volunteer efforts and the long hours logged by Lori, as well as myself, my sister, Jessica, my brother, Alex, and others, we've been able to train mental health practitioners in the community to use tapping with their trauma patients. "They've really been amazing," Lori says of the work that group of 24 has since been able to do in Newtown. We've all also done tapping with kids, administrators, health-care professionals, as well as teachers who were touched by this terrible tragedy. There are an estimated 10,000 adults and children within the Newtown school community, and the healing work we are doing with them continues. "This town is healing," Lori shares. "Something extraordinary is possible here, but it's going to take some time."

In its first 18 months, the foundation has not only had a huge impact in Newtown; its work has quickly spread beyond the town's borders. Lori, who's now the director of the foundation, has also been working remotely with groups that survived natural disasters and trauma in Oklahoma, Arizona, the Philippines, and Liberia. The foundation has also done work with businesses, including a program with the New York Department of Transportation.

The sheer number of requests for support that are pouring into the foundation has grown exponentially. "It's more than I can manage on my own right now, due to funding," Lori explains, "but the growth is phenomenal, and we're working on a pilot program for schools that's about to go global. It's really, really exciting to see how far we've come in just a year and a half."

Lori adds, "I see miracles everywhere, and we've experienced so many miracles in how things came together here in Newtown, and now in other parts of the U.S. and around the world. Really, everything's possible at this point. We call ourselves the Emotional Red Cross. It's just incredibly rewarding work."

Personally, for me, it's been the most fulfilling work of my adult life. I've known for a long time that tapping was extraordinarily effective in healing trauma and The Tapping Solution Foundation had been supporting work around the world for several years, but never did I imagine that I would be doing this work so close to home. I feel honored to be able to play a part in helping Newtown heal and in spreading this important message around the world to those who need it most.

To watch some of the incredibly inspiring work Lori and the foundation are doing in Newtown and around the world, visit tappingsolutionfoundation.org.

Is there something you'd love to do but haven't yet done? A cause you'd love to support, a hobby you'd love to turn into a business, a skill you've always wanted to learn, or a place you've always yearned to travel to? Can you imagine yourself actually doing it? If there's one thing I've learned from starting this foundation and doing the tapping work I do, it's that the world desperately needs each of us to contribute our talents and live our lives in the most authentic way possible. Whatever it is you've been yearning to do, start taking baby steps every day toward realizing those dreams. If you keep moving forward, you'll be amazed by what you can both accomplish and contribute.

BIBLIOGRAPHY

"AAPM Facts and Figures on Pain." The American Academy of Pain Medicine. http://www.painmed.org/patientcenter/facts_on_pain.aspx.

"About Chronic Pain." Stanford Systems Neuroscience and Pain Lab. http://snapl.stanford.edu/research/about-chronic-pain.

Bakalar, Nicholas. "Back Pain Remains Overtreated." *The New York Times* (August 2, 2013).

Beecher, Henry K. "Relationship of Significance of Wound to Pain Experienced." *Journal of the American Medicine Association (JAMA)* 161, no. 17 (August 1956): 1609–1613. http://jama.jamanetwork.com/article.aspx?articleid=323093.

"The Brain, Pain and Personal Finance." EarthSky Podcasts published by PBS Learning Media. http://www.pbslearningmedia.org/resource/db18cb58-ff2d-48e1-b814-1cb0bfa1e36f/db18cb58-ff2d-48e1-b814-1cb0bfa1e36f.

Brown, Brené. "3 Ways to Set Boundaries." *Oprah*. http://www.oprah.com/spirit/how-to-set-boundaries-brene-browns-advice.

Church, Dawson. "Clinical EFT as an Evidence-Based Practice for the Treatment of Psychological and Physiological Conditions." *Scientific Research* 4, no. 8 (August 2013). http://www.scirp.org/journal/PaperDownload.aspx?paperID=35751.

Clark, David. D. *They Can't Find Anything Wrong!* Boulder, CO: Sentient Publications, 2007.

"Complex Regional Pain Syndrome Fact Sheet." NINDS. NIH Publication No. 13-4173 (June 2013). http://www.ninds.nih.gov/disorders/reflex_sympathetic_dystrophy/detail_reflex_sympathetic_dystrophy.htm.

Craig, Gary. *Emotional Freedom Techniques for Back Pain*. Fulton, CA: Energy Psychology Press, 2009.

Ephraim, P. L., et al. "Phantom Pain, Residual Limb Pain, and Back Pain in Amputees: Results of a National Survey." *Archives of Physical Medicine and Rehabilitation* 86, no. 10 (October 2005): 1910–1919. http://www.ncbi.nlm.nih.gov/pubmed/16213230.

Goodwin, R. D., and M. B. Stein. "Association Between Childhood Trauma and Physical Disorders among Adults in the United States." *Psychological Medicine* 34, no. 3 (April 2004): 509–20. http//www.ncbi.nlm.nih.gov/pubmed/15259836.

Hanson, Rick. *Hardwiring Happiness*. New York: Harmony Books, 2013.

Keller, A., et al. "Does the Perception That Stress Affects Health Matter? The Association with Health and Mortality." *Health Psychology* 31, no. 5 (September 2012): 677–684. http//www.ncbi.nlm.nih.gov/pubmed/22201278.

Klein, Stefan. *The Science of Happiness*. New York: Avalon Publishing Group, 2006.

Lipton, Bruce H. *The Biology of Belief*. Carlsbad, CA: Hay House, 2008.

"Low Back Pain Fact Sheet." NINDS. NIH Publication No. 03-5161 (July 2003). http://www.ninds.nih.gov/disorders/backpain/detail_backpain.htm.

Maldarelli, Claire. "Is the Brain Hard-Wired for Pain?" *Scienceline* (November 4, 2013). http://scienceline.org/2013/11/is-the-brain-hard-wired-for-pain.

Maté, Gabor. *When the Body Says No*. Hoboken, NJ: John Wiley & Sons, 2003.

Mercola, Joseph. "Another Study Finds Arthroscopic Knee Surgery No Better Than Sham Surgery." Mercola.com. http://articles.mercola.com/sites/articles/archive/2014/02/07/arthroscopic-knee-surgery.aspx

Moffet Jennifer, Kalber, et al. "Randomised Controlled Trial of Exercise for Low Back Pain: Clinical Outcomes, Costs, and Preferences." *BMJ* 319, no. 7205 (July 1999): 279–283. http://dx.doi.org/10.1136/bmj.319.7205.279.

Neighmond, Patti, and Richard Knox. "Pain in the Back? Exercise May Help You Learn Not to Feel It." NPR (January 13, 2014). http://www.npr.org/blogs/health/2014/01/13/255457090/pain-in-the-back-exercise-may-help-you-learn-not-to-feel-it.

"New CT Scans Reveal Acupuncture Points." *HealthCMi* (January 4, 2014). http://www.healthcmi.com/Acupuncture-Continuing-Education-News/1230-new-ct-scans-reveal-acupuncture-points.

O'Connor, Anahad. "Acupuncture Provides True Pain Relief in Study." *The New York Times* (September 11, 2012). http://well.blogs.nytimes.com/2012/09/11/acupuncture-provides-true-pain-relief-in-study/?_r=0.

"Pain: Hope Through Research." NINDS. NIH Publication No. 01-2406 (December 2001). http://www.ninds.nih.gov/disorders/chronic_pain/detail_chronic_pain.htm.

Pert, Candace B. *The Molecules of Emotion.* New York: Scribner, 1997.

Reynolds, Gretchen. "Doctors Identify a New Knee Ligament." *The New York Times* (November 13, 2013).

Sanders, Luke. "Anatomical Structure Discovered for Acupuncture Points." *Health Acupuncture* (January 5, 2014). http://www.healthacupuncture.co.uk/research/anatomical-structure-discovered-for-acupuncture-points.html.

Sarno, John E. *Healing Back Pain.* New York: Warner Books, 1991.

———. *The Mindbody Prescription.* New York: Warner Books, 1998.

Schubiner, Howard, and Michael Betzold. *Unlearn Your Pain: A 28-Day Process to Reprogram Your Brain.* Pleasant Ridge, MI: Mind Body Publishing, 2010.

"The Science of Pain." *UC Davis Medicine* (Fall 2007). http://www.ucdmc.ucdavis.edu /ucdavismedicine/issues/fall2007/features/8.html.

Smith, Michael. "Negative Emotions Increase Pain." *Medpage Today* (September 27, 2010). http:/www.medpagetoday.com/Rheumatology/Fibromyalgia/22431.

Whitbourne, Susan Krauss. "The Complete Guide to Understanding Your Emotions." *Psychology Today* (May 19, 2012). http://www.psychologytoday.com/blog/fulfillment-any -age/201205/the-complete-guide-understanding-your-emotions.

White, Donna M. "4 Tips for Setting Healthy Boundaries." Psych Central. http://psych-central.com/blog/archives/2013/08/17/4-tips-for-setting-healthy-boundaries.

Younger, Jarred, et al. "Viewing Pictures of a Romantic Partner Reduces Experimental Pain: Involvement of Neural Reward Systems." *PLoS ONE* 5, no. 10 (October 2010). http:// www.plosone.org/article/info%3Adoi%2F10.1371%2Fjournal.pone.0013309.

INDEX

ACKNOWLEDGMENTS

The amazing people in my life are what made this book possible, in so many ways. To my wonderful wife, Brenna, who makes me laugh every day and makes sure I don't take anything too seriously. Alex and Jess, it just keeps getting funner and funner, and we're changing lives together (yeah, I know that's not a word, but I'm thinking I can get away without edits in this part of the book . . .). Mom and Dad, you really are the kindest, most patient, wisest parents anyone could ask for, though I'm sure I didn't feel that way when I was 13. Karen, Malakai, Lucas, Olivia, Penny, the first reader of my first book, the Taylors, and especially Alison Taylor, whose life goal is to see her name printed in as many languages as possible (you're welcome), and so much other amazing family. Much love to you all.

Erin Walrath—I cherish our friendship and the fact that it survived me forgetting to mention you in the acknowledgments of my first book. That's a real friendship. Peter Mariano, you might as well make a cameo here. Nick Polizzi and Kevin Gianni, I am grateful on a daily basis for our friendship, the great times we have, and the mutual support. Kris Carr, thanks for your friendship, business advice, and incredible support every step of the way. And congratulations on the amazing job you did in "Un Argentino en Nueva York"—truly your best work. (YouTube it if you're a Kris Carr fan and curious . . .)

To the amazing family at Hay House, because it truly is a family. Patty, thank you for believing in me and this work. Reid, it's an honor to work with such a

213

brilliant man on so many different levels—thanks for your faith and support. Nancy, I cherish our times together at I Can Do Its and look forward to many more. Laura, thanks for being such a steady hand on this book. And, of course, Louise Hay, who made all of this possible and continues to be a bright light in the world—thanks for your friendship, for making me laugh, and for being such a shining example of how to live and love.

To Wyndham Wood—it is truly a pleasure and an honor to work with you so closely on this book. You're brilliant and I'm so grateful to have you in my life. Thank you, thank you. To Mary Ayers and Michelle Polizzi, thanks so much for your help on this book.

To Lori Leyden—thank you for the incredible work you've done and continue to do with The Tapping Solution Foundation. Our greatest accomplishments are yet to come!

To my friends in the tapping and personal development community: Eric Robins, thank you for the wonderful foreword; Wayne Dyer, Cheryl Richardson, Mark Hyman, Lissa Rankin, Carol Look, Lindsey Kenny, Tim Ryan, Mike Dooley, Dawson Church, David Feinstein, Stacey Vornbrock, thanks for your incredible contributions to the world and to this book.

To the Tapping Solution Team, thank you for all your support and hard work on getting this important message out to the world.

To all the people who have opened their hearts to my coaching and have contributed their experiences to this book, I've been transformed in helping you change! To the hundreds of thousands of people on my e-mail list: though I know very few of you personally, I am touched by your support and your commitment to yourself and to the world.

To the foundation upon which my work stands, the incredible innovations and breakthroughs made by Roger Callahan, Gary Craig, and Pat Carrington. Without you, none of this would be possible!

And last, to the person (hopefully not plural . . .) I inevitably forgot in these acknowledgments. My advance apologies and I'll make it up to you in the next book!

ABOUT THE AUTHOR

Nick Ortner is the creator and executive producer of the hit documentary film *The Tapping Solution* and author of the *New York Times* best-selling book *The Tapping Solution*. He has also produced the annual worldwide online event the Tapping World Summit, which has been attended by more than one million people.

Ortner is a dynamic speaker, presenting breakthrough live tapping sessions around the world, consulting with companies and organizations on how to integrate EFT Tapping and stress-relief techniques, and working to spread the use of tapping in schools, hospitals, and other organizations. He lives in Newtown, Connecticut. Follow Nick on Twitter @nickortner and see him on Facebook at facebook.com/nortner

EXTRA RESOURCES

If you're looking to take your tapping experience to the next level, we have a variety of resources available on multiple subjects:

The Tapping Solution Free E-mail Newsletter: Get weekly content and stay up to date on the latest in EFT Tapping by signing up here: www.thetappingsolution.com.

Dive Deeper in Your Pain Relief Journey: Watch an interactive webinar on pain relief and receive more pain relief resources here: www.thetappingsolution.com/painbook.

Losing Weight and Letting Go of Fear, Guilt, and Shame around Food: Download a free tapping meditation designed to help you lose weight (normally sold for $19.95 but free to all purchasers of this book) at www.thetappingsolution.com/weightloss.

Creating Love and Healthy Relationships: Manifest the love you desire or improve your existing relationship here: www.thetappingsolution.com/love.

Making Money and Achieving Your Dreams: Download a free tapping meditation to relieve financial stress and anxiety and create a more abundant life (normally sold for $19.95 but free to all purchasers of this book) at www.thetappingsolution.com/money.

Hay House Titles of Related Interest

YOU CAN HEAL YOUR LIFE, the movie, starring Louise Hay & Friends
(available as an online streaming video)
www.LouiseHayMovie.com

THE SHIFT, the movie, starring Dr. Wayne W. Dyer
(available as an online streaming video)
www.DyerMovie.com

THE BIOLOGY OF BELIEF:
Unleashing the Power of Consciousness, Matter & Miracles,
by Bruce H. Lipton, Ph.D.

MIND OVER MEDICINE:
Scientific Proof That You Can Heal Yourself,
by Lissa Rankin, M.D.

THE TAPPING SOLUTION FOR WEIGHT LOSS & BODY CONFIDENCE: A Woman's Guide to
Stressing Less, Weighing Less, and Loving More,
by Jessica Ortner

YOU ARE THE PLACEBO:
Making Your Mind Matter,
by Dr. Joe Dispenza

All of the above are available at your local bookstore,
or may be ordered by contacting Hay House (see next page).

We hope you enjoyed this Hay House book. If you'd like to receive our online catalog featuring additional information on Hay House books and products, or if you'd like to find out more about the Hay Foundation, please contact:

Hay House, Inc., P.O. Box 5100, Carlsbad, CA 92018-5100
(760) 431-7695 or (800) 654-5126
(760) 431-6948 (fax) or (800) 650-5115 (fax)
www.hayhouse.com® • www.hayfoundation.org

———

Published in Australia by: Hay House Australia Pty. Ltd.,
18/36 Ralph St., Alexandria NSW 2015
Phone: 612-9669-4299 • *Fax:* 612-9669-4144
www.hayhouse.com.au

Published in the United Kingdom by: Hay House UK, Ltd.,
The Sixth Floor, Watson House, 54 Baker Street, London W1U 7BU
Phone: +44 (0)20 3927 7290 • *Fax:* +44 (0)20 3927 7291
www.hayhouse.co.uk

Published in India by: Hay House Publishers India,
Muskaan Complex, Plot No. 3, B-2, Vasant Kunj, New Delhi 110 070
Phone: 91-11-4176-1620 • *Fax:* 91-11-4176-1630
www.hayhouse.co.in

———

Access New Knowledge.
Anytime. Anywhere.

Learn and evolve at your own pace
with the world's leading experts.

www.hayhouseU.com